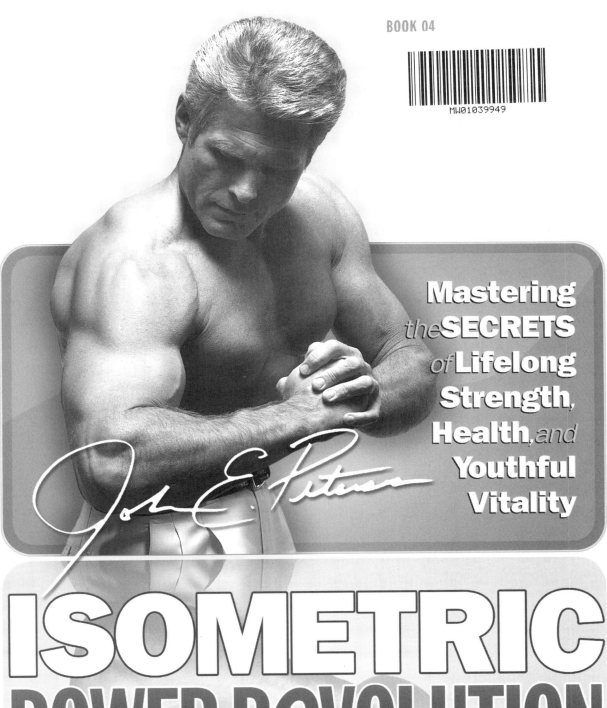

BOOK 04

Mastering *the* **SECRETS** *of* **Lifelong Strength,** **Health,** *and* **Youthful Vitality**

ISOMETRIC POWER REVOLUTION

JOHN e. PETERSON

author of *Pushing Yourself to Power* and *The Miracle Seven*

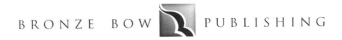

BRONZE BOW PUBLISHING

Dedicated to the memory of Isaac Neal Eslinger.
Where we saw great promise, God saw perfection.
·January 27, 2005 — September 19, 2005

ISOMETRIC POWER ReVOLUTION

Most of the photos in the history chapter
are courtesy of Sandow & the Golden Age of Iron Men.

ISBN-13: 978-1-932458-50-3; ISBN-10: 1-932458-50-6

Published by Bronze Bow Publishing, Inc.
2600 E. 26th Street, Minneapolis, MN 55406.

You can reach us on the Internet at www.bronzebowpublishing.com

Literary development and cover/interior design by
Koechel Peterson & Associates, Inc., Minneapolis, Minnesota.

Manufactured in the United States of America

TABLE of CONTENTS

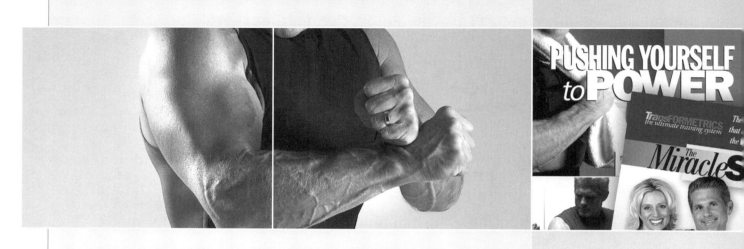

INTRODUCTION

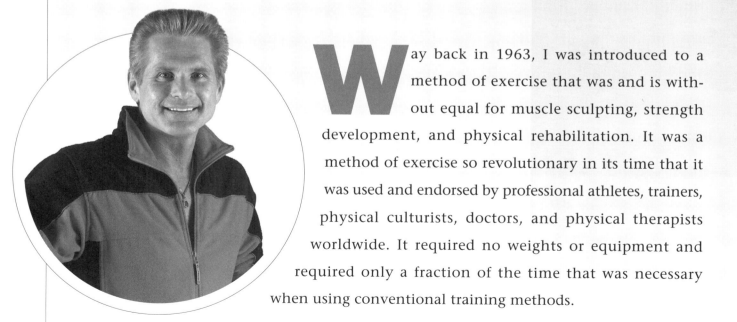

Way back in 1963, I was introduced to a method of exercise that was and is without equal for muscle sculpting, strength development, and physical rehabilitation. It was a method of exercise so revolutionary in its time that it was used and endorsed by professional athletes, trainers, physical culturists, doctors, and physical therapists worldwide. It required no weights or equipment and required only a fraction of the time that was necessary when using conventional training methods.

Most important of all, this method of exercise had been verified scientifically in hundreds of experiments conducted with more than 5,000 volunteer test subjects at the Max Planck Institute in Dortmund, Germany under the direction of Dr. E. A. Müeller and Dr. Theodore Hettinger between 1946 and 1961. The results of their experiments and research were astounding. When compared to all other methods of exercises, in *every* case this method of exercise was proven vastly superior for the acquisition of muscular strength, and it was also proven to be the safest. As a result, this method was used

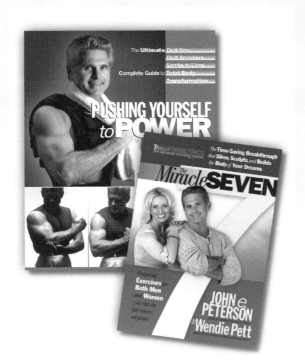

extensively in physical rehabilitation by medical researchers and therapists on a worldwide scale.

Intrigued? You should be.

This is how I described my introduction to this incredible method of exercise in my second book, *The Miracle Seven*:

66 The first time I saw an Isometric Contraction properly performed was in July 1963, when I was ten years old. It was about a month after my grandfather and Uncle Wally took me under their wing and put me on the Charles Atlas Dynamic Tension Training System. The occasion was the annual family reunion, which was always a great time. And, of course, even though I had only been training for a month, Uncle Wally and Grandpa were already telling everyone about how much muscle I had built in only 30 days. (Nobody ever had anyone more affirmative in their life than my grandfather and Uncle Wally were for me. They were like two guardian angels. I hope some of you men realize what a profound impact you can have in a boy's life if you just take the time to notice and affirm them.)

The family reunion was a magical day. My dad and uncles were just getting going on their World War II stories when Uncle Milo showed up. Milo was the tallest of my uncles— he was 6'3" and weighed 210 pounds of the most perfectly sculpted muscle you could possibly imagine. But somehow he looked different that day. Now keep in my mind that my grandfather had put all six of his sons on the Charles Atlas Training System as soon as they reached twelve years of age, *if not* sooner, and all the brothers had exceptional physiques. They all looked like living, breathing Greek statues.

It was my dad who spoke up. "My gosh, Milo, what have you been doing? You look like someone carved you out of stone."

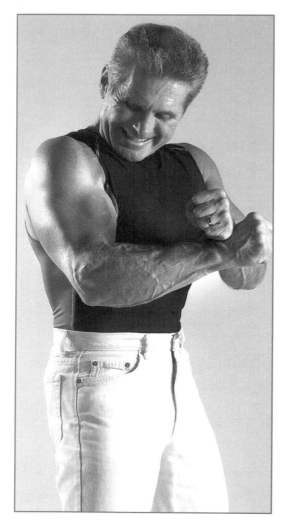

When I heard Dad say that, I did a double take. It was true. Uncle Milo's facial and neck muscles were even

more obvious than usual, and his forearms were sheer cords of muscle.

"Well, Al," said Uncle Milo, "I started adding Isometrics to my Dynamic Tension Exercises about four months ago, and everyone tells me that they can see a big difference."

Believe me, you could. Then all my uncles as well as my grandfather started talking about Isometrics. As it turned out, Milo started practicing Isometrics after he read an article about President Kennedy practicing them on the advice of the White House physicians. Milo reasoned that an Isometric exercise was really a Charles Atlas self-resistance exercise where so much force was applied in both directions that no movement occurred because the muscles were involved in a deadlock wrestling match against each other for 10 seconds.

"Exactly how do you do that, Milo?" my uncle Robert asked.

Uncle Milo stood up and took off his shirt. To this day I have never seen a more perfectly developed man. I've seen lots of guys with bigger arms, bigger chests, and bigger legs, but I've never seen one more perfectly put together than my uncle. In fact, if you've ever seen the physique of the actor Woody Strode, you know precisely what my uncle Milo looked like.

Well, Milo did a few self-resistance Atlas biceps exercises to warm his muscles up and then on the fourth rep, halfway up he performed an Isometric Contraction. With all his might, his left arm was pushing down while his right arm was pulling up. For 10 seconds his muscles looked as though they were involved in a life-or-death struggle. Far more than just a biceps Isometric Contraction, it appeared as though every muscle in his entire body was flexed to its absolute limit. Literally, every muscle fiber in his neck, pectorals, arms, abs, and back stood out in bold relief. It was an incredible demonstration of how to perform an Isometric Contraction correctly.

When Uncle Milo finished, my grandfather said, "That's how the strongman Zass trained. Same kind of exercises I read about years ago in *Physical Culture,* but I'd never actually seen it done until now."

Seriously, if you had seen my uncle perform that Isometric Contraction on that day, you'd never wonder whether or not Isometric Contraction is a valuable form of exercise. No, instead you'd be standing in line to buy the course and learn how to do it. **"**

And that, my friend, leads us to this book, *Isometric Power Revolution.* Why? Because this book IS that course my uncle Milo should have written back in 1963. I hope you enjoy it.

John E. Peterson, January 2007

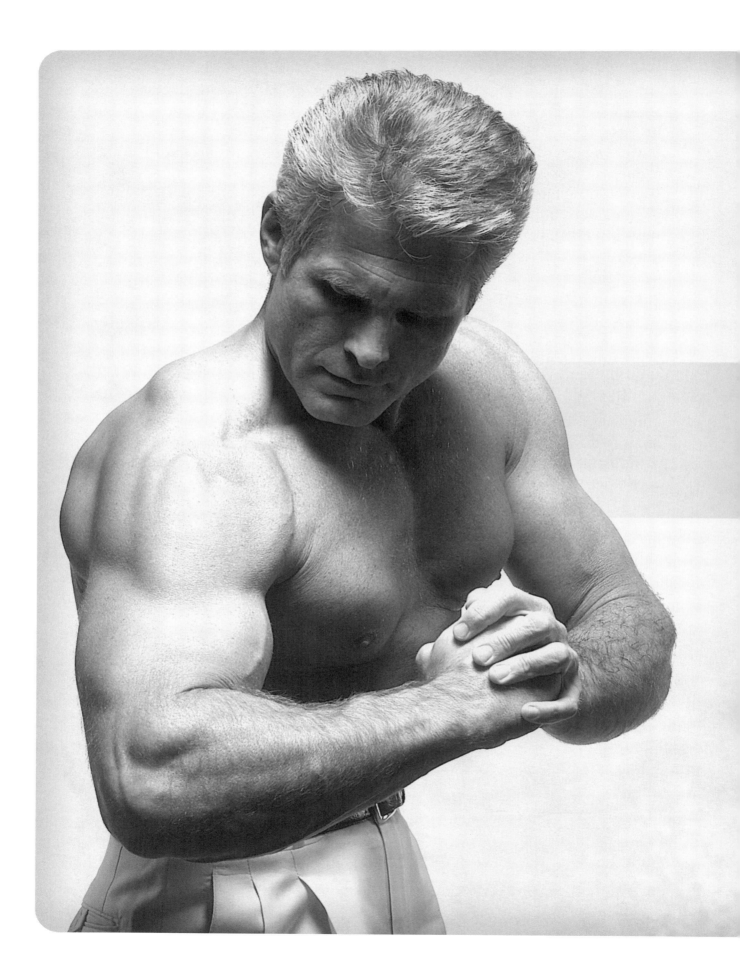

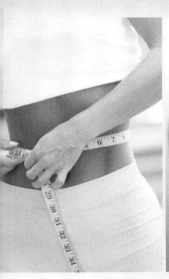
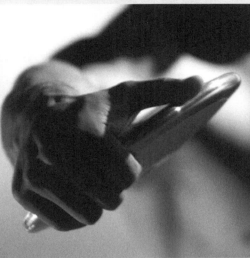
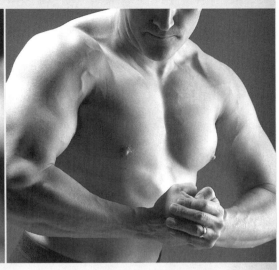

BEGIN *with the* **GOAL** *in* MIND

The Master Key to Success With Isometric
Contraction and Everything Else in Life

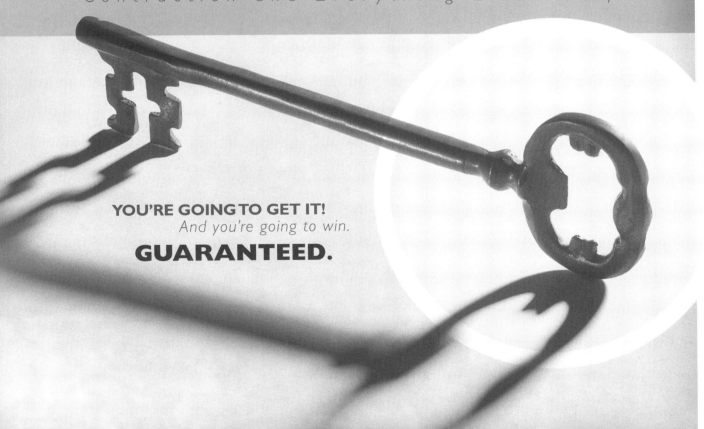

YOU'RE GOING TO GET IT!
And you're going to win.
GUARANTEED.

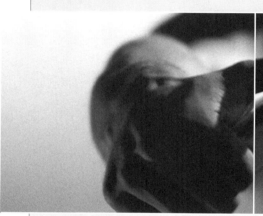
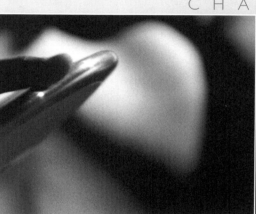
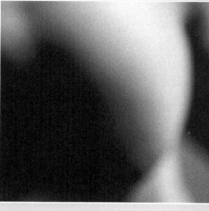

BEGIN *with the* GOAL *in* MIND

*The Master Key to Success With Isometric
Contraction and Everything Else in Life*

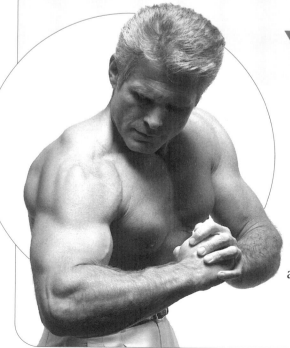

Your success with our Isometric Power program is predicated on following the instructions presented in this book to the letter. A failure to heed or comprehend this introductory information or to think that it is unessential fluff or that you already know it is almost certain to short-circuit the program's effectiveness. The Master Key to Isometric Contraction, perhaps more than any other exercise program, begins with the most important exercise in existence, and about which most people are completely ignorant.

That Master Key is:

1. **Programming the right thoughts into your mind.**

2. **Focusing on them.**

3. **Actualizing them by following through.**

Think about it: you would not have invested in this Isometric Power course if you weren't influenced by the thoughts you were consciously thinking at the time you bought it. Likewise, you will not take action to give yourself the supreme state of health, strength, and lifelong fitness that you desire and *deserve*, unless you begin with the goal, the end result, clearly defined in your mind. Don't try to prove me wrong on this point by underestimating the power of your mind, as you'll only end up shortchanging yourself.

Let's be real. Most people think that strength and fitness success is nothing more than a combination of knowing the right exercises and eating the right foods. Although that is definitely *part* of the route to success, the truth is that you cannot get the results you want, much less stick with the right exercises and nutrition program, unless your mind is programmed properly.

Take a look around, my friend. There are hundreds of thousands of people who pay expensive gym memberships, exercise and diet year after year, and they are still overweight and lacking in muscle definition. They go through the motions, but they don't get anywhere. *Why is that?* Because they don't understand the

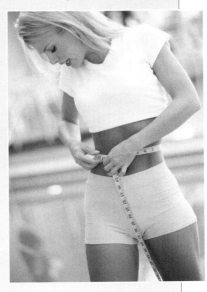

life-changing power that God has placed within them. Even worse, when introduced to it, they flat out reject it. They are literally afraid to take control of their own thinking mechanism. Truth to tell, these people fear that any attempt to harness their mind will backfire. Instead of boldly living the life of their dreams, they timidly settle for whatever life hands them. They want someone else to give them the answers, and that, my friend, is not only sad, it's living by default.

This is not the way of the Transformed life, and it continually is not the way of any Transformetrics™ student or practitioner. You, and you alone, will determine what you want in life—and you alone, with faith, courage, and perseverance, will make up your mind that nothing will prevent you from reaching your goal. You're going to get it! And you're going to win. Guaranteed.

YOU'RE GOING TO GET IT!
And you're going to win.
GUARANTEED.

The keys to achieving this Transformation in consciousness that attracts success and repels failure in all facets of your life are not difficult to learn. And they don't require a lot of time. Just follow my step-by-step instructions, and you will be on the fast track to success in no time flat.

ISOMETRIC POWER BREATHING

Let's start with Isometric Power Breathing. Why Isometric Power Breathing? Here are three reasons:

1. **Breath is the source of life. Breath is power. Breath is life.**

2. **Deep breathing calms, centers, and focuses the mind so that you can better comprehend what you're about to learn in the following chapters.**

3. **Deep breathing puts you into an awakened state of awareness in which you not only think clearly but realize that you can create the life you have dreamed of living.**

Whether or not you are a Bible-believing Christian, if you will just take a moment to read the creation story as found in the first two chapters of the Book of Genesis, you will find something fascinating. First of all, whenever God created something, it states clearly that He pictured it in His mind first. Second, after God created the first man, the man did not come to life until...

"And the LORD God formed man of the dust of the ground, *and breathed into his nostrils the breath of life*; and man became a living soul" (Genesis 2:7 KJV, emphasis mine).

I'm telling you this because the whole key to making miracles happen in your life begins the exact same way. First, you establish order through mentally picturing what it is that you want to achieve. Then you add power, life, vitality, radiance, and passion to the mental image by breathing life into it.

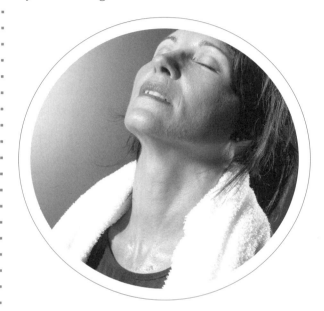

The good news is that this process isn't difficult to learn. Not only that, but the deep breathing method you're about to learn will simultaneously accomplish a number of things that I know you will be excited about. Instead of telling you exactly what they are in advance, let's go over the exercise.

HOW TO PERFORM ISOMETRIC POWER BREATHING:

1. **In the morning, before arising from your bed, lie on our back and relax with your hands at your sides.**

2. **Inhale deeply through your nostrils and imagine that you are filling your entire body right down to your toes with**

enriched oxygen. Literally, let yourself expand.

3. Once you can inhale no farther, hold for a count of 7 seconds, while pulling in your abdominal muscles, then begin to exhale.

4. During the exhale, squeeze your abdominal muscles as though you are wringing water from a wet towel. Squeeze the entire rectus abdominus from top to bottom as tightly as possible, while making an *"sssss"* or *"fffff"* sound.

5. When you have achieved peak intensity or contraction of the abdominals, hold for 7 or more seconds, squeezing until your exhale is completely finished. Leave nothing in your lungs. Try to get everything out.

6. While performing step 5, it is a healthy practice to contract or pull your perineum up and inward. This will not only improve your overall energy, but greatly improve sexual function as well.

7. Perform this Isometric Power Breathing exercise 10 times in succession before getting out of bed. You are then welcome to get up, stand before an open window, and do more of the same. You can also do this exercise anytime throughout the day to release mental stress and to recharge and energize

yourself. Just remember to consciously flex your abdominals when performing this exercise.

Now that you have read the instructions, put the book down and take a few minutes to perform this breathing technique 10 times. In order to get you fired up and motivated about this, and just in case you missed some of the benefits in the steps outlined above, here is a recap of the many benefits of practicing this breathing technique:

- **Increases mental clarity and alertness.**
- **Enhances creative and mental power.**
- **Rids your entire body and mind of negative stress.**
- **Strengthens, tightens, and tones the diaphragm and entire abdominal muscle structure. Some people lose inches of fat from their abdomens.**
- **Improves digestion and elimination.**
- **Cleans the lungs of stale residue.**
- **Helps you relax.**
- **Improves dynamic strength and power due to strengthening of core muscles.**

All these benefits come from just one set of Isometric Power Breathing exercises. Enough said. So get to it and complete 10 repetitions. Feel for yourself just how powerful Isometric Power Breathing truly is.

Okay, great. Once you've completed your set of 10 power breaths, you will be feeling energized, and, simply put, you should feel *good* all over. That *good feeling* is the *Golden Key* to success in life, especially when you learn to harness it and combine it with the mental programming techniques that you will learn here.

MORE THAN JUST THINKING

The bottom line is that we don't just become what we think about, as King Solomon said, "As a man thinketh in his heart, so is he." We become what we think about with deep, vivid emotion. To merely think a thought does not give it transformative power. But to think a thought backed by an abundance of passion, enthusiasm, and positive, life-affirming emotion puts it into the realm of the extraordinary. And when that happens, it's "look out world," because here you come.

Note: we think in pictures. For example, think of your children or spouse. What comes to mind? A picture, right? Now think of your home, your car, your television, your favorite restaurant, your church, and so on. What do you see in your mind's eye? One picture after another, correct? Remember that. Our thoughts are pictures.

Our thoughts are literally what we envision. And what does *envision* mean? It means to see the outcome as reality *before* it happens, in our mind's eye. This is crucial for you to understand, and it is the *mental tool* you need to achieve your greatest desire. That desire might be for a powerful, perfectly sculpted body and radiant health, or it can be for anything else you want to create in your life.

Since this is a book about how to give yourself radiant health, strength, and the kind of body you have always dreamed of having, I want you to form a mental picture of the kind of fitness and type of physique you want to have. Do you want to dramatically enhance the size of your muscles? Or do you want to achieve a lithe, lean, ripped look of a gymnast? Or something in between. Whatever your choice, it can be achieved with the Isometric Power methods outlined in this book.

Not so sure about that? Take a look at the photos of Dr. Neal Eslinger, Mark Baldwin, Chris Rezny, and our other friends featured within the pages of this book. They all achieved their dreams by following the methods outlined here and modifying them to fit their own personal goals, and you can too!

In one sense, this is no different from other forms of bodybuilding. Some people train to get huge, and others to get lean. But what most people *erroneously* assume is that they achieve their goals merely by the choice of physical exercise itself. Truth to tell, you don't! For instance, you could practice all the classic power lifts or Olympic lifts and not gain an ounce of weight. It's done all the time.

So what then is the Golden Key to gaining muscle and losing fat with an exercise program? Simply put, *the key is your intention.* What is it you want? What do you see in your mind's eye? C'mon, picture it. Tell your muscles how you want them to respond to the exercises, and they will obey.

Your flesh has an intelligence (you'll read all about it in the history section), and it simply sits back and waits for you to give it orders. Once the orders are given and systematically applied, every cell in your body goes to work to shape your body the way you want it.

THE POWER OF YOUR THOUGHTS

For this reason, it is imperative that you never ever . . . not under any circumstances . . . allow yourself to think or say anything about yourself that you do not wish to be absolutely true. That's how powerful your thoughts and mental imagery are.

We know that it is possible for some people who are sick to make themselves well by choosing the right thoughts to think. We also know from medical science that the exact opposite can happen by thinking negatively. It happens every day in every city throughout the world. Consider the following true case history that I shared in my first book, *Pushing Yourself to Power.* It

clearly communicates the power of our thoughts to create our reality.

In an article published in 1957 by psychologist Bruno Klopfer in *The Journal of Prospective Techniques,* a man named Mr. Wright suffered from advanced lymphatic cancer. His lymph nodes were swollen to the size of oranges, and both his spleen and liver were so enlarged that two quarts of milky fluid had to be drained from them daily. The doctors had done everything medically possible in the mid 1950s on Mr. Wright's behalf, and there was nothing more they could do. So they gave him up to die.

Somehow Mr. Wright heard of a new experimental drug for cancer. But it was only being administered to people whom doctors believed had at least a three-month life expectancy. Wright begged his doctor for the drug, and finally the doctor relented. According to the report, the doctor injected him on Friday but really didn't expect him to live through the weekend. Unbelievably, on the following

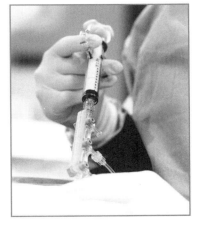

Monday, less than 72 hours later, Wright was walking around and feeling great. The tumors, according to the article, had "melted like snowballs on a hot stove." Ten days after his first Krebiozen injection, Mr. Wright went home from the hospital, being determined by the doctors to be cancer free!

Unfortunately, months later the American Medical Association published a nationwide study on Krebiozen that flatly announced it was worthless. Mr. Wright read the study, believed it, and his cancer returned. Two days later he died.

So what happened to Mr. Wright? Why did he become wrong? Let's examine it objectively. Mr. Wright, who is terminal, hears about a new miracle cure for cancer. He reasons to himself that the reason he has not already died is because it is his destiny to be cured of cancer and Krebiozen is the agent of that cure. He begs his doctor to go outside the rule and inject him. Then Mr. Wright's intellect and emotions, his mind, *believes* that the miraculous cure has been found, and as a result his body obeys the single congruent message that it is given by Mr. Wright's mind, which is—HEAL! And his body has no other choice but to obey!

Just think what would have happened had Mr. Wright not read the study that negated his positive belief. Who knows how long he could have lived? The simple point is this: whatever you believe about yourself, both intellectually and emotionally, will determine who and what you become physically and spiritually. For that reason alone, you must guard your thoughts, your speech, and all of your associations. If you surround yourself with positive reinforcement in what you see, hear, think, and verbalize, and if you follow through with positive action—you will meet with a positive outcome. It is inevitable!

YOU MUST BELIEVE

Do you get the point? Your mind, your beliefs, your faith, all determine what you can have or be. *If you don't believe you can have or be something, you won't.*

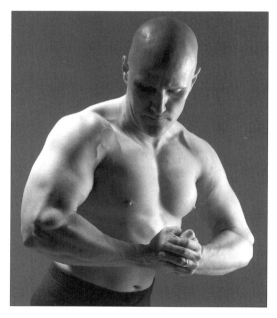

This applies to your strength and fitness as much as it does to any other facet of your life. Dr. Neal Eslinger, whom you see pictured throughout the Iso Powerflex section of this course wanted to accomplish two things simultaneously. He wanted to get ripped and lean while adding muscle mass. Look at his before and after photos (on page 135)—same man in both photos. The fact that he simultaneously achieved the lithe, ripped look while adding greatly to his muscle mass is mind-boggling for most people. How did he do it?

First and foremost, he wanted to do so. Second, by forming a clear picture in his mind's eye of exactly *what* he wanted to achieve and thinking about it all the time. Third, by holding the exact image in mind while he trained. It's as simple as that.

The unrevealed *secret* that most people never discover is not just picturing what they want, but picturing it with passion and conviction. Put some white heat behind your desire, and you cannot help but go in the direction of your dreams. This is a universal law. Whatever dominates your thoughts and passions is what you become. Guaranteed.

HOW TO APPLY POSITIVE EMOTION TO YOUR GOAL

It's very simple to learn to use your emotions to help reach your goals.

To demonstrate this, I want you to use Isometric Power Breathing. First, perform your standard 10 Isometric Power Breaths, concentrating on your abdominal muscles as you did previously. Next, before starting your next set of Isometric Power Breaths, I want you to consciously form a mental picture in your mind's eye of what you want to achieve while inhaling. Quite literally, I want you to surround this mental image with breath. Instead of focusing on your abdominal muscles, focus on the mental imagery and add self-talk to it as you squeeze (add passion and emotion) to

the mental image. Then, after you have completed your inhale, begin your exhale. But instead of just breathing out, maintain a laser-like focus surrounding your mental image with the emotion-backed energy. Literally, exhale and breathe life into the image, surrounding it with power. Do it 10 times.

Understand that there is a reason why the great sages of all times throughout history practiced deep breathing exercises while in prayer and meditation. And the same can be done before anything creative is attempted. Whether painting, drawing, writing, singing, or public speaking, breathe deep to center yourself and take control. It all starts with your breath.

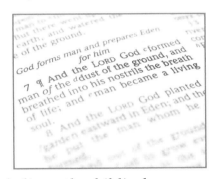

Think back to the creation story as told in the Book of Genesis. Remember the key that I mentioned earlier? God breathed life into Adam. Whether or not you personally believe the biblical account of creation is *not* my point. My point is that the process of creation as described in Genesis is exactly what you want to use in your life. Always remember that you are not just a man or a woman—you are a human being created in the very likeness of God with a divine thought and creative ability that is literally molded after God. Consider this: if man was created in the image and likeness of God, and God is the Preeminent Creator, then it makes perfect sense that man is also intended to be a creator...and is at his happiest and most God-like when he too is creating.

This is why clearly defined goals are so important. We are happiest when we are creating. We are less than happy, if not downright miserable, when we are not creating. So form a goal and add life to it through Isometric Power Breathing and visualization. Begin and end every workout with deep Isometric Power Breathing. Never begin a creative endeavor of any sort without taking a few minutes to perform 10 Isometric Power Breaths.

Will it change the outcome? Big time.

SOAR LIKE AN EAGLE

Before you close this chapter, you must perform a couple of written exercises that are vitally important to your personal success. *Do Not Overlook These.* If you want to soar like an eagle, play close attention and follow through.

Many people, in fact most people, when asked to define what it is they want in life literally draw a blank. They can't clearly articulate what they want because their minds have been so preoccupied with what they *don't* want for so long that it appears that there is nothing else for them.

So what can we do? We already know that we become what we habitually think about with deep emotion. And so, if you can't even think about what you want because you have so much thought and energy invested in what you don't want,

guess what you are creating? You got it. MORE of what you DON'T want.

So does that mean that you are doomed to a life of mediocrity and unfulfilled dreams? Only if you blow this off and don't take positive action. It's only too late if you don't start now!

Seriously, my friend, there is a way out of any bottomless pit of despair. So let me guide you with a brief writing exercise that could change your life. But before you make a list of what you want, I want you to make a list of everything you despise and don't want.

Take out a pad of paper and a pen and write this headline across the top of the page: *Things I Don't Want and That I Will Eliminate From My Life.*

Now, beneath this headline start writing those things that come to your mind. Don't worry about perfect grammar. Just list everything in your life that you consider a source of personal embarrassment or self-sabotage. For example:

- **I don't want to be fat.**
- **I don't want to be weak.**
- **I don't want to be out of breath from walking up a flight of stairs.**
- **I don't want any more back pain.**
- **I don't want these headaches.**
- **I don't want to buy clothes at Huge and Huger.**
- **I don't want women or men to look away when they see me.**
- **I don't want to be passed over in job promotions by fitter people. (Don't kid yourself, it happens all the time.)**
- **I don't want my children to be ashamed to be seen with me.**
- **I don't want to be afraid to be seen in a swimsuit.**
- **I don't want to be afraid to train in public.**

Get the idea? Good. Then get to it. Do it now before you do anything else.

The only rule concerning what you write is that it must be something you want to change. So please. Do it now. Don't move until you've done this. Put your pen to the paper and write out everything that has held you back and that you want to eliminate from your life. If you run out of space, get another piece of paper and keep writing. After all, it's your life that you're going to heal.

Congratulations! It takes guts to face yourself and tell yourself the truth about what you are no longer willing to accept because you know in your heart of hearts that God created you for so much more.

SO WHAT DO YOU WANT IN LIFE?

Now that you have identified what you don't want, your mind will be clear and uncluttered. That being true, right now is also the time to identify what you do want in life. So let's get to it.

Keep in mind that you can write anything on this list that you want. It doesn't all have to be strength and fitness related. But then again, the stronger, fitter, more vibrant, and self-confident you are, the easier it will be to have every other good thing on your list.

So here's what you do. On a clean sheet of paper, write the headline: *The Good Things That I Want to Create in My Life.* You'll want to list at least 10 things that you want to achieve within the next 12 months. For example, your list may include some of the following:

- **I want to double my strength.**
- **I want to see my abdominal muscles in the mirror.**
- **I want my kids to be proud to be seen with me.**
- **I want to have all my pants taken in at the waistline.**
- **I want people to compliment me on my new physique.**
- **I want my boss and business associates to view me as**

someone with guts, determination, and a *get it done—no excuses* drive that deserves a big promotion.

- **I want to buy $100 worth of Girl Scout cookies to give to the food shelf in my community.**
- **I want to attract the perfect mate in my life.**
- **I want to double my current income.**

Okay, you know what to do, so do it. Don't be afraid to dream big because small dreams have no power. After all, at this point you deserve all the best that life has to offer. So do it now.

Great job!

Now that you have identified what you want, you can always go back and add precise details. The more clear and vivid the details the better the result. The key, however, is to take the time to identify what you want and put it down on paper.

CHOOSING ONE GOAL

After you have completed your two lists, it's time to focus on just one goal. This goal needs to be something that is achievable within the next 30 days. In fact, it may even be something you achieve in just 7 days. If you don't have a short-term goal, then take a few minutes and come up with one. It's crucial that you do it. Why? Because I want you to prove to yourself that you can set goals and achieve them. Doing so will build personal

confidence quickly. Once you know that you can focus on a goal and make it happen, your creative power will grow by leaps and bounds, and you will gain the confidence to achieve bigger and bigger goals at faster and faster rates.

So this is what you do. Select one goal that you will focus on. Write it on a 3" X 5" card and give it a deadline for accomplishment. For example, you might write the following:

"By _____, exactly 31 days from now, I will do 50 consecutive Tiger Stretch Push-ups in flawless form." Or it can be anything else that you want.

Now, each day when you awake, focus on this goal during your deep breathing exercises. Perform 10 Isometric Power Breaths while focusing on your abdominals and applying Isometric Contraction on both inhalation and exhalation. Then do another 10, focusing entirely on your goal as previously directed. Put passion, enthusiasm, and determination into it, and breathe life into the image in your mind's eye.

Next, carry the 3" X 5" card with you everywhere you go. Make it easily accessible—put it in your front pocket, your wallet, tape it to the refrigerator, or wherever. Take it out and read it several times a day with *deep conviction*.

Then when you do your exercises, visualize achieving your goal. Notice the laser-like focus that you now have and how much harder you train. Most importantly, notice how quickly you improve!

While you train, tell yourself, "I can. I will. I can. I will."

Then add the ending to it, "I can and I will do 50 consecutive Tiger Stretch Push-ups by _____."

After you have achieved your goal, I want you to say out loud, "I can. I will. And I've done 50 consecutive Tiger Stretch Push-ups." At this point, write the accomplishment and date of completion on your goal card and save it. It is important that you begin a collection of completed goal cards, because in the future it will reinforce your ability to get things done when you review them.

BEYOND YOUR WILDEST DREAMS

What I have just revealed is the Master Key to achieving anything you want in your life. You could join the vast hosts of people who spend thousands of dollars attending personal empowerment seminars to learn what I have just revealed to you. If you implement this Master Key into your life, you can achieve goals that are beyond your wildest dreams. Without it, you can achieve very little. Why? Because you need to know where you are going in order to get there. And that applies to every facet of your life, including your strength and fitness.

In my opinion, this first chapter is the most important of all. Why? Because anyone can teach you Isometric exercises. Anyone can teach a diet to follow. But the whole key that makes any of it work lies within you. When you control your thoughts, you control your life. And, truth to tell, your ability to think and persevere is the key to achieving superior results with Isometric Contraction or anything else in your life.

Now that you know the secret, let me fill you in on "The History of Isometric Contraction," and why I believe it is singularly the Master method to lifelong strength and fitness. Read on.

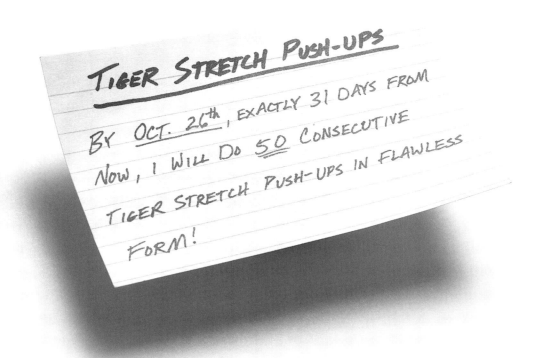

TIGER STRETCH PUSH-UPS

BY OCT. 26th, EXACTLY 31 DAYS FROM NOW, I WILL DO 50 CONSECUTIVE TIGER STRETCH PUSH-UPS IN FLAWLESS FORM!

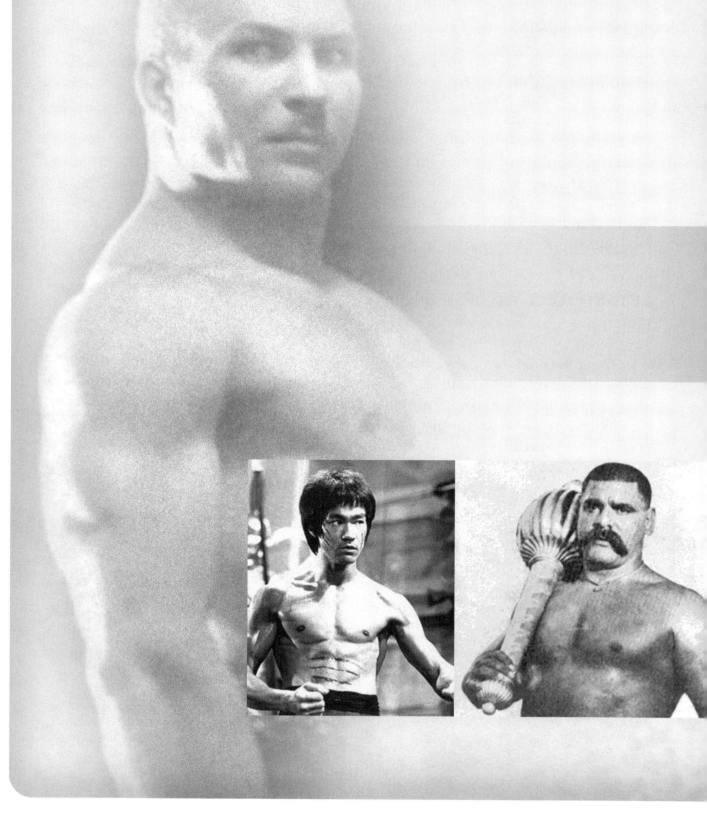

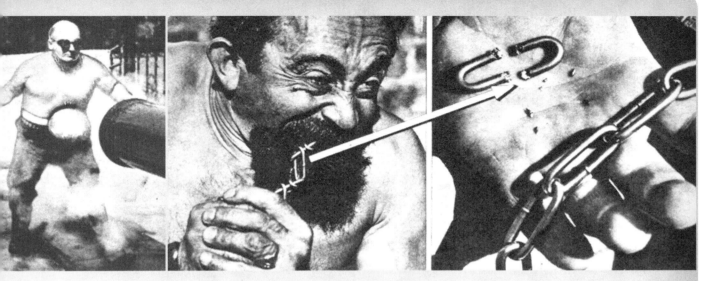

a **CONCISE HISTORY**
of ISOMETRIC CONTRACTION

NOTE: *If you are not interested in the history of Isometric Contraction, read this chapter anyway, because you will be, and you should not deny yourself the sheer pleasure you'll get from it.*

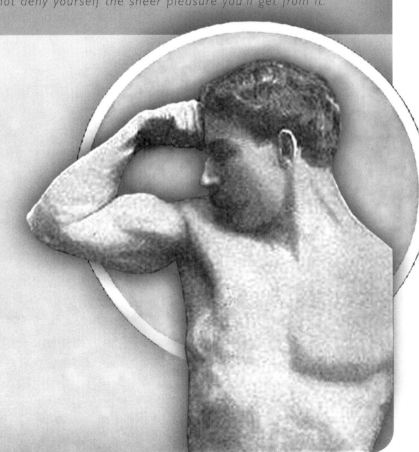

"What has been will be again, what has been done will be done again; there is nothing new under the sun."

—Ecclesiastes 1:9

TWO

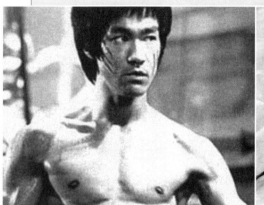 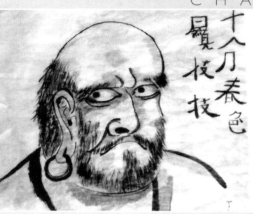 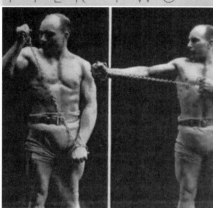

a CONCISE HISTORY *of* ISOMETRIC CONTRACTION

Since ancient times, mankind has been fascinated with the acquisition and development of exceptional physical strength. After all, who hasn't heard of the renowned biblical heroes Samson and King David? Or the Greek hero Hercules? Or King Odysseus, the famed Greek hero of Homer's *The Odyssey*?

All of these men were known for their extraordinary strength, intellect, and courage. And if you read their stories closely, you'll discover that King David, Hercules, and

King Odysseus all had one thing in common—their ability to both string and pull to full draw *a bow made of bronze*. Twice in the Bible, for instance, King David states: "He *trains* my hands for war, so that *my arms can bend a bow of bronze*" (Psalm 18:34; 2 Samuel 22:35). Notice that David was trained and strengthened in this feat of strength. But that's not the only time a bronze bow was referred to in antiquity.

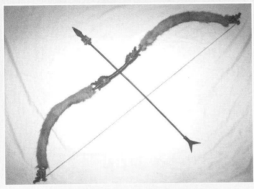

A replica of the "bow of bronze"

In fact, if you read *The Odyssey*, you'll find that the Bronze Bow of Hercules plays a central role (almost a character-like role within the story) in King Odysseus's reclaiming his wife and kingdom of Ithaca from suitors who are trying to steal his kingdom. At the climax of the story, Odysseus proves that he, and he alone, can string and pull to full draw the Bow of Hercules and send an arrow through 12 small consecutively placed brass rings without touching any of them. This is precisely what he had done some 20 years earlier on the day he won the hand of his wife, Penelope, in marriage by proving himself to be the best man physically as well as intellectually. After the sheer precision with the rings, King Odysseus uses his archery skills to fend off the suitors.

Similar to King David, Odysseus did not just pick up Hercules' Bronze Bow and pull it to full draw. Hercules had befriended the young Odysseus when they were sailing together as crew members with Jason and the Argonauts on the ship Argo to discover the fabled Golden Fleece at the edge of the world. According to the story, Hercules taught the secrets of strength to Odysseus. His training was so effective that, besides Hercules, only young Odysseus could string and pull to full draw an arrow on the famed Bronze Bow of Hercules. That's all I'm going to tell you about it. If you want to know more…and there is more…read the stories of David and Odysseus for yourself and strengthen your mind.

So what does a bronze bow have to do with Isometrics in a chapter devoted to the histories of Isometric Contraction? Good question. The answer lies in reading the accounts of any number of historians of the ancient past, such as Herodotus (often known as the father of history) and his anecdotal *History*, which includes a description of the war between the Greeks and Persians in the fifth century B.C., or Josephus and his *Antiquities of the Jews,* or Plutarch's *Parallel Lives* from the first century. In their writings, you will discover that archers were considered to be the elite special forces of their day and among the strongest and fittest of ancient warriors.

So how did archers achieve this status? Well, consider the fact that many of the battles of ancient history were determined by the army that had the strongest and most accurate archers. For instance, if one army's archers were capable of picking off their enemy's soldiers at a distance 200 yards farther away than the enemy's archers, it gave that army a decided advantage. Consequently, it was the archers alone who oftentimes determined the outcome of a major battle in ancient times. Such was the case at the Battle of Marathon in 490 B.C., where the heavily outnumbered Greeks defeated the Persians. This was also the case in the battle between the Syrians and the Israelites as recorded in 1 Kings 22:29 in the Bible. Here a Syrian archer determined the outcome of the battle when he killed King Ahab of Israel.

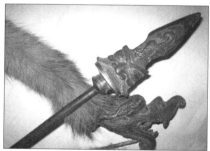

A close-up of a bronze bow and arrow

The importance of ancient archers relates to the history of Isometric Contraction as several ancient historians, and especially Herodotus, commented on the training of the archers. This is how it was done. First, there was a selection process to determine which individuals had the innate skills to become a first-class archer. This included tests of hand/eye coordination, eagle-like sight, and uncanny depth perception. The other critical attribute was superb physical strength, as demonstrated in the ability to hold an arrow at full draw, sometimes for extended periods of time.

This is where Isometric Contraction comes into place. The ancient trainers would have a trainee pull back the strongest bow of which he was capable and then hold it—an Isometric Contraction. The trainee would continue this practice until he could finally draw the arrow to full draw with ease. At this point, the trainee would graduate to a heavier bow and draw it back as far as he possibly could and once again hold it in an Isometric Contraction. When he could draw it back with ease, the archer graduated to an even heavier bow and continued the strengthening process by reapplying Isometric Contraction. This training process was continued until each archer achieved the ability to draw the strongest of bows, a process that often required years, and Isometric Contraction was the key.

INDIA AND THE ORIENT

In a very real sense, Isometric Contraction is among the oldest of exercise methods known to man. It has been a part of hatha yoga (the physical branch of the popular form of yoga that most Westerners are familiar with) for almost 5,000 years. It has developed primarily in southern India by ascetics who led very disciplined lives. They lived close to the earth and observed nature, animals, and themselves. These ascetics would imitate many of the animals they observed—their postures and habits—in order to emulate their strength, grace, and wisdom.

From this intense study, hatha yoga developed into a complex series of postures and poses (well over 1,000 in all) called "asanas" that require incredible levels of strength, flexibility, muscular endurance, balance, coordination, deep synchronized meditative breathing, and an intense mind/muscle connection.

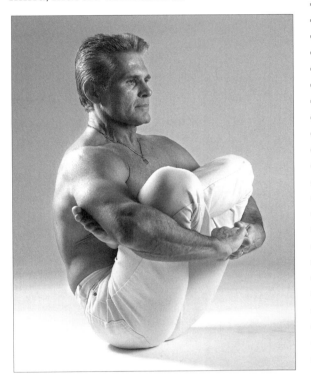

As an example, study the pose shown in the photo above. Now, imagine yourself trying to hold this pose for 3 minutes without shaking or quivering. What type of strength would you need to develop in order to hold that pose in picture-perfect alignment? In a word: *Isometric.* Let me explain why. The word *Isometric* comes from the Greek (what else would you expect?) word *iso,* meaning "the same," and *metric,* meaning "length." *Isometric Contraction* refers, therefore, to the contraction or tightening of a muscle without changing its length, which is exactly what you are doing when *holding* yoga poses such as the one pictured here. (If, for any reason, you don't think this requires incredible concentration and strength, then put the book down and try to hold the pose shown for 3 minutes. If by some miracle you can hold it, please tell me why you bought this book.)

As is clearly evident, it is Isometric Contraction alone that allows you to maintain these postures by stabilizing the entire muscle structure. Is it tough? You bet it is, but you wouldn't be developing the epitome of strength and poise if it weren't.

ISOMETRICS IN THE ORIENT

Somewhere between A.D. 500 and 527, legendary Buddhist Master Bodhidharma traveled from India to China to bring Chan Buddhism to the monks of the Shaolin Temple. He was said to be an extraordinary man in every sense of the word, and one of the strongest, fittest, and wisest men to have ever lived. Traveling by foot and alone, he crossed raging streams and rivers, a major part of the Himalayan mountain chain, and braved extremes of temperature ranging from tropical rainforest heat to subzero cold in some of the tallest mountains on planet earth.

As if that were not enough of a test of his fortitude, Bodhidharma also exposed himself to the dangers posed by wild animals and mountain bandits. In other words, this was not a trip you'd want to take without a group of guardian angels watching your every move. Yet, this is exactly what the missionary of Chan Buddhism took upon himself to do.

Upon his arrival at the original Shaolin Temple on Mount Song in northern China's Henan Province, Bodhidharma did not find a group of "Kwai Chang Caine" look-a-likes from the TV series *Kung Fu,* who could "snatch a pebble from my hand" as young Grasshopper would often attempt to do with the blind Shaolin monk "Master Po." Nor did he find anyone who even remotely resembled the perfectly sculpted supermen of the Shaolin monk movies that so many of us have seen, featuring the likes of Bruce Lee, Jackie Chan, or Jet Li. No, the guys whom he found were so fat and out of shape they couldn't even stay awake for the rigors of prayer and meditation that he was to teach them.

So the first thing he did was to leave the temple and spend the next nine years meditating in a cave in order to figure out what to do. When he returned, he used his skills as a yoga master to teach the monks a series of special exercises of his own creation that are still practiced in martial arts training systems to this very day. And what were these special strengthening exercises that transformed the sheepish monks of the Shaolin monastery into the Warrior Monks of Legend (as they came to be known) whom nobody in their right mind wanted to mess with?

Believe it or not, they were exercises that

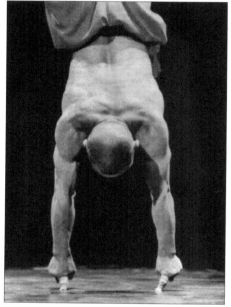

Only Isometrics can develop the tendon strength in the fingers for this incredible feat of strength.

had a very strong Isometric component in them. In fact, it is believed that the "I Chin Ching" or "Yi Jin Jing" or Muscle/Tendon Changing Classic was one of the original forms taught by Bodhidharma himself. This form includes the use of deep breathing exercises, which should be a part of every strength and conditioning program, combined with Isometric muscle contractions of the hands and arms. Amazingly, this Isometric form was and is so effective that it has remained virtually unchanged for approximately 1,500 years.

In addition to the Isometric forms of Bodhidharma, there are also numerous dance-like katas or forms found in other Asian martial arts that include various Isometric postures that are often held for extended periods of time just as in hatha yoga from which they originate. Some of these postures include the "Iron Wire" form of hung gar kung fu and sanchin kata of Okinawan martial arts systems. Of course, there are different names used in the various martial art forms that reflect the countries and cultures from which they originate, but ultimately it all boils down to the same concepts of holding deep stances against the pull of gravity for long periods of time and using ultra-high tension strength building techniques that are Isometric in nature.

ISOMETRICS IN WARFARE

As you can imagine, Isometric Contraction as a strength training method has also been utilized in just about every culture throughout the centuries. For instance, the chariot racers of ancient Rome pulled against the reins of their horses for extended periods of time, which is a powerful Isometric Contraction. As you might imagine, the charioteers were incredibly strong men.

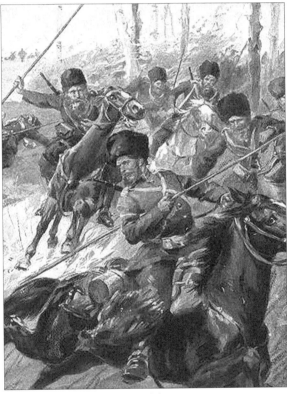

Russian Cossack horsemen

The same is also true for mounted cavalry. The French army led by Napoleon Bonaparte was literally vanquished by Russian Cossack horsemen who were capable of doing amazing feats at a full gallop. Consider that when Napoleon marched into Moscow in 1812, he had 465,000 troops. The Cossacks were a mere fraction of that number. And though the Cossacks refused to engage Napoleon's army on the open field of battle, they nonetheless earned both the respect and fear of the surviving French soldiers. According to the historians' accounts of the experiences of the soldiers who survived Napoleon's retreat, the Cossacks would attack at all hours of the day and night. Their favorite targets were supply wagons and artillery batteries, often jumping tremendous barriers on horseback and lopping off the heads of the enemy without breaking stride.

The Cossacks were similar to the Mongol horsemen of Genghis Khan (five centuries earlier), who were capable of shooting large numbers of arrows at full gallop. The Cossacks appeared to move with their horses as though rider and horse were one being. Their athleticism on horseback was something to behold. Even the French soldiers couldn't help but admire it. In reality, it was because of the superior strength and conditioning of the leg muscles that they had developed that allowed the Cossacks to perform these astounding feats.

So what type of strength do you suppose will keep you in the saddle or on horseback under virtually any conditions? You got it. *Isometrics.*

As an interesting matter of historical fact, the Cossacks chased Napoleon's forces all the way to the gates of Paris. Less than 40,000 survivors of Napoleon's Grand Army (*La Grande Armée*) of 465,000 men lived to tell about the retreat from Moscow, and in 1814 the Cossacks were present in Paris when Napoleon was forced to abdicate and unconditionally surrender and was subsequently exiled to the Italian island of Elba. To this very day, there is one surviving Cossack word that remains a part of the French language—*bistro*. Today it means "a bar or roadside restaurant," but back in 1814 it was used by the Cossacks when they put their rubles down on the bar and said, "Bistro," which meant *be quick about it*.

ISOMETRICS IN POPULAR LITERATURE

In 1844, *The Count of Monte Christo* was published by Alexander Dumas. Its hero, Edmond Dantès, was a handsome, promising young sailor with a beautiful fiancée named Mercédès and a bright future with a commission as a ship's captain. But then he is a victim of conspiracy of four jealous and unsavory characters who arrange to have him seized and secretly imprisoned in solitary confinement in the infamous Château d'If, a dangerous offshore prison from which no one had ever escaped. For many years, Dantès barely exists in his tiny isolated cell. He almost loses his mind and his will to live as his body slowly weakens, deteriorates, and becomes emaciated.

Then one day Dantès hears a fellow prisoner burrowing nearby. He too begins digging, and soon he meets an old abbé (a lower-ranking Catholic clergyman). From the abbé, Dantès learns history, literature, science, ancient and modern languages,

and the secrets of strengthening and conditioning his body for the incredible task that lies ahead of him to make good his escape from the Château d'If. It is here that many references are made to strengthening exercises that had to be Isometric in nature. Throughout the balance of the novel, there are numerous references to the count's extraordinary physical strength and prowess. And as you can imagine, this novel also inspired many other men to try similar exercises for strengthening their bodies, such as Alexander Zass, whom you'll meet later on in this chapter.

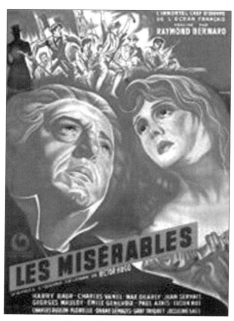

Les Misérables poster

Victor Hugo's *Les Misérables* is another novel that makes reference to Isometric type exercises, and it also deals with a man who was imprisoned. It was originally published in France in 1862 and tells the story of Jean Valjean and his amazing struggle to not only become a free man but a saintly one—a man who has been fully redeemed by God's grace in every sense of the word. Throughout the references to Jean Valjean's time of imprisonment, there are many references to his extraordinary physical strength. For instance, the following paragraph is taken word for word from page 90, and it makes a direct reference to Isometric strength building exercises:

> "His suppleness even exceeded his vigor. Some convicts, who perpetually dream of escaping, eventually make a real science of combined skill and strength; it is *the science of the muscles. A full course of mysterious statics is daily practiced by the prisoners,* those eternal enviers of flies and birds. Swarming up a perpendicular, and finding a resting place where a projection is scarcely visible, was child's play to Jean Valjean. Given a corner of a wall, with the *tension* of his back and hams, with his elbows and heels clinging to the rough stone, he could hoist himself as if by magic to a third story, and at times would ascend to the very roof of the bagne."

Of course, there are several other references in various novels and books to Isometric strength building exercises. In his 1970 autobiography *Papillon*, Henri Charrière often refers to his *static* Isometric exercises that made his muscles feel like iron when he was incarcerated in a penal colony on French Guiana in the 1930s and 1940s. In fact, these exercises helped him survive his time in solitary confinement, where he did not hear a single word from another human being for more than two years. Charrière is the only man to ever escape from Devil's Island, which is located off the coast of French Guiana.

As you can see, from the ancients to the moderns, Isometric Contraction has been a part of history and literature for millenniums of time. Still, the science behind Isometric Contraction was not validated until the twentieth century.

ISOMETRICS AND THE GOLDEN AGE OF PHYSICAL CULTURE

In a very real sense, the Golden Age of Isometric Contraction coincided with the Golden Age of Physical Culture, which began with the dawning of the twentieth century. During this time, the Industrial Revolution was taking hold in America, and large numbers of people were moving from an agrarian farming lifestyle to an industrial and more urban one. As a result, more and more people were using their mental capacities rather than their physical capacities to earn a livelihood. Correspondingly, more people began suffering from the diseases of modern life that are caused by too much of the wrong kinds of food and too little of the right kinds of exercise. That is reflected in the fact that a male born in 1900 had a life expectancy of just 47 years and a female of just 49 years. Bottom line: *these weren't the good old days—not by a long shot.*

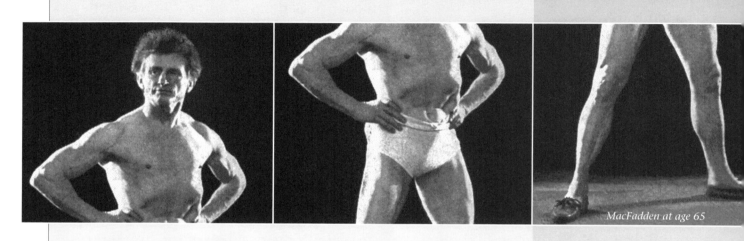

MacFadden at age 65

BERNARR MACFADDEN
. . . .
" T h e   F a t h e r   o f   P h y s i c a l   C u l t u r e "

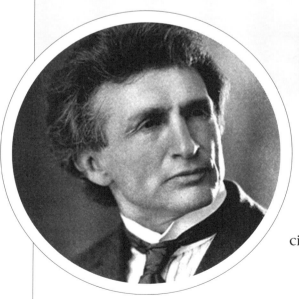

n March 1899, a young man in his early 30s with a passion for physical fitness and exercise came into prominence when he published his first issue of *Physical Culture* magazine. This publisher's name was Bernarr MacFadden, and in just four years his slogan "Weakness Is a Crime, Don't Be a Criminal" had resonated so well with an ever-growing audience in America that *Physical Culture* magazine reached a monthly circulation of more than 100,000 copies.

But MacFadden didn't limit himself to being a magazine publisher only. In 1906, he published his own natural bodybuilding book, *Muscular Power and Beauty,* which featured photos of MacFadden teaching a complete system of self-resistance and Isometric exercises for every muscle group in the body. He was so convinced of the superiority of his Isometric/self-resistance methods that on the title page of his book he wrote:

> " Containing detailed instructions for the development of the external muscular system to its utmost degree of perfection. "

The truth was, when you saw the photos of MacFadden's flawless physique as he demonstrated the exercises, it made it impossible to argue with the effectiveness of his methods. The man clearly knew what he was talking about and was the "living proof personified." Believe me, when it came to weakness, Bernarr MacFadden was no criminal.

For more than 40 years, MacFadden's *Physical Culture* magazine had an avid audience that reached into the hundreds of thousands. In both 1921 and 1922, the Golden Years of Physical Culture Magazines, MacFadden had two contests to determine America's most perfectly developed man. The winner of both contests was a young man who trained with the exact same methods that were found in MacFadden's *Muscular Power and Beauty*. Though he discovered the methods in another source, the man's name was Charles Atlas, who became the stuff of legends.

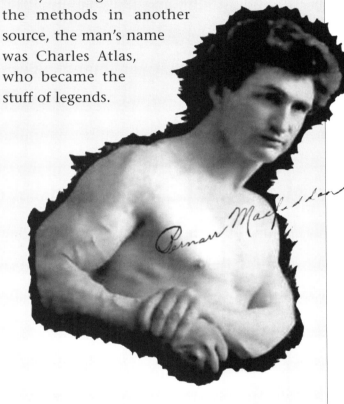

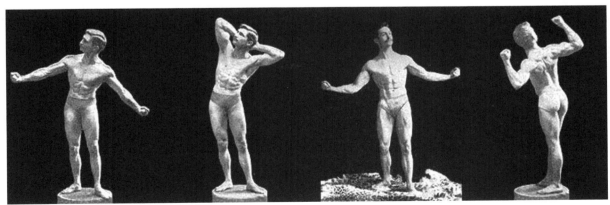

MacFadden classical poses

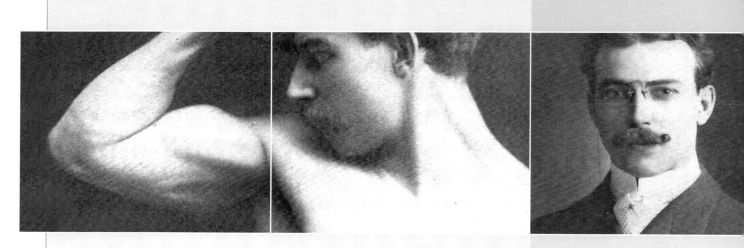

ALOIS P. SWOBODA

"The Father of Conscious Evolution"

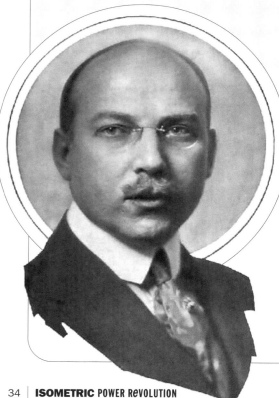

At approximately the same time that MacFadden began teaching his methods of self-development, there was another equally famous physical culturist, Alois P. Swoboda, who also taught a system that required no apparatus of any kind. He was so certain of the incredible benefits of his exercise system that he stated in his advertising copy: "By this condensed system more exercise and benefit can be obtained in ten minutes than by any other in two hours." His ads usually featured his perfectly developed Greek-godlike physique in one photo at the top right of the page and another photo usually at the bottom left of the page, where he appeared to be a well-dressed, cultured, successful, and exceedingly handsome aristocratic gentleman.

The fact that Swoboda appealed to men from across the spectrum of society is clearly evident. Among his students were President Theodore Roosevelt, two members of the Supreme Court, doctors, lawyers, and athletes of all types, the magician Harry Houdini, as well as ranch hands, miners, and lumberjacks. Swoboda also had an incredible array of testimonials. Truth to tell, in all respects the man was brilliant, and his knowledge of anatomy and physiology was second to none. In a very real sense, Swoboda was more than a century ahead of his time. Take, for example, his explanation of the dangers of lifting heavy weights and why his system of physiological exercise was vastly superior.

❝ First, I desire to say that physiological exercise produces health and strength and improves one's physique.

A system of exercise to be physiological must not produce these results at the expense of the heart, arteries, or vitality. Now, then, it is a fact that the use of heavy weights is a speedy route to development, because of the resistance they give to the muscles; but they cause an enlargement and dilation of the heart and also produce aneurism, on account of the obstruction they give to the circulation of the blood in the capillary blood vessels. The capillaries lie in between the muscular fibers, and as the latter contract they shorten and necessarily widen, consequently compressing anything that lies between them, hence the obstruction of the circulation of the blood in the capillaries.

Since heavy weights cause a continual contraction of the muscular fibers while they are being used, it is readily seen that there is a constant obstruction to the circulation. And since the heart is constantly forcing blood into the arteries, and it cannot empty into the capillaries and pass into the veins, there is a great increase of pressure in the arteries, which reacts on the heart and causes hypertrophy of that organ.

Therefore, since heavy weights cause a rapid development of muscle and strength by means of the resistance they give, it is a fact that by offering the muscles the same resistance (which is done by using one muscle to resist or antagonize another), one will receive the same development. And since heavy weights overtax the heart and arteries by the constant obstruction they cause, it is also a fact that by making the contraction intermittent by means of alternate relaxations, the circulation of the blood will not be obstructed, but, on the contrary, with each relaxation, the blood will flow from the arteries into the capillaries, and each

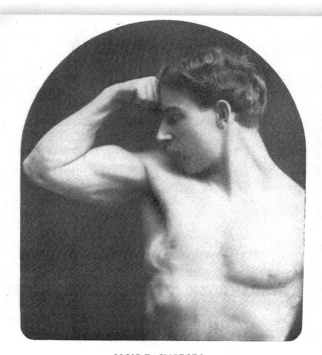

ALOIS P. SWOBODA.
Originator and Instructor of the Only Scientific and Physiological
Method of Exercise.

The Swoboda System of Physiological Exercise.

(From the Boston Post)

THE NEWEST WAY TO ATTAIN PERFECT HEALTH.

Alois P. Swoboda Antagonizes Two Sets of Muscles with Phenomenal
Results.

Alois P. Swoboda has discovered a way by which, through antag-
onization of the muscles, a person may become as strong as he
likes, and all this without artificial aid. While at nineteen years of
age he was looked upon as a consumptive, to-day his chest and
abdominal muscles are so strong that he can uphold a thousand
pound weight upon them.

This remarkable state of affairs is the result of a brand new
system of development, the secret of which is told in the preceding
paragraph. In the accompanying statement, over his own signature,
Mr. Swoboda details some very interesting facts. While not posing
as a strong man in the sense usually given that word, Swoboda has
given some examples of his strength which easily place him among
the first of the men of muscle. For instance, he will take a pack of
cards and tear it into two pieces; then he will tear the halves into
quarters, and the quarters into eighths, using but his thumbs and
fingers. He will do the same thing with two packs.

This is by no means all. He will first raise a 275-pound dumb-
bell over his head. Then he raises a 200-pound dumb-bell over his
head six times in succession without letting it down. He has raised
a two-pound dumb-bell 6,000 times in 53 minutes and 20 seconds.

Here is his own story:

"When nineteen years of age, I was very weak and debilitated.
The fact that my father died of consumption five years previous, and
the warning of my friends that I would follow the same route, caused
me to look toward exercise as a means of building up my health and
strength. I began the study of anatomy for the location, functions
and relations of all the muscles. I studied physiology to find the
physiological effect of exercise; why exercise caused development,
and the effect of different modes of exercise. I soon found that the use of heavy weights was the speediest route to development. But
I also found that the use of the weights checked the capillary circu-
lation, thereby increasing the pressure in the arteries, consequently
placing an undue strain on the heart. Since, however, the use of
weights caused a rapid development of the muscles and will power
and at the same time overtaxed the heart, it occurred to me that if I
could find a means by which the muscles could be offered the same
resistance as by the use of weights (and still not use weights), that I
could gain as much muscle, will power and vital force in as short a
time, and not overtax the heart, which is unavoidable when weights
are used.

"In studying anatomy I soon noticed that while all movable parts
of the body had muscles to move them one way, they also had muscles
to move them back again. It then occurred to me that to use one
muscle to offer resistance to another would cause the same development as the use of weights to offer resistance, but with the alternate
contractions and relaxations, would help the venous circulation and
instead of obstructing the circulation in the capillaries, would help
the blood in the course towards the heart, thereby resting the heart.
Therefore, the alternate contractions and relaxations of one muscle
under the influence of a stimulus (will power) to antagonize another
is the principle of my system of physiological exercise.

ALOIS P. SWOBODA."

SWOBODA'S MEASUREMENTS.

BEGINNING.	AFTER THREE YEARS.
Chest, normal, 34 inches.	Chest, normal, 45 inches.
Chest, contracted, 33 inches.	Chest, contracted, 34 inches.
Chest, expanded, 35½ inches, showing an expansion of the chest of 2½ inches.	Chest, expanded, 52 inches, showing an expansion of 18 inches.
Waist, 31 inches.	Waist, 29 inches.
Neck, 13¾ inches.	Neck, 16½ inches.
Biceps, 11⅞ inches.	Biceps, 16 inches.
Forearm, 10⅞ inches.	Forearm, 13¼ inches.
Thigh, 18½ inches.	Thigh, 24 inches.
Calf, 13 inches.	Calf, 15 inches.
Weight, 130 pounds.	Weight, 160 pounds.

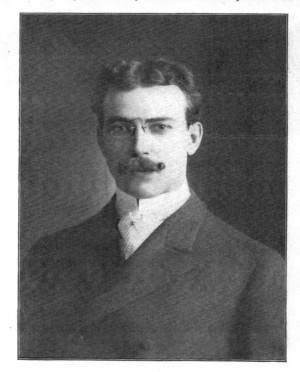

ALOIS P. SWOBODA.

57 Washington St.,   Chicago, Ill.

contraction will force it from the capillaries into the veins and help it in its course toward the heart."

Swoboda wrote this *more than a century ago* in his Swobodaism Course, which he copyrighted in 1901. The exact same dangers that Swoboda mentions were completely verified by today's medical establishment and revealed to the public in an article published in the March 13, 2003 issue of the *Wall Street Journal* titled "Fears Mount Over Dangers of Pumping Iron: Weightlifting Craze Comes Under Scrutiny by Doctors Concerned About Health Risks." When I say that Swoboda warned of the exact dangers that have now been verified by medical science, I'm not saying *similar* to—I'm saying *exact*. You can read the *Wall Street Journal* article on line for yourself.

So what exactly did Swoboda teach his students? I have seen a copy of the original Swoboda course, and his exercises were a combination of ultra-high tension Isometric Power Flexes (similar to the ones featured in this book) followed immediately by a movement where the tension in the muscles was reduced just enough to permit movement through a complete range of movement while the muscles remained under intense contraction. This was followed by a *complete relaxation* of the effected muscle groups between repetitions that allowed the blood to flow unimpeded as mentioned in the previously quoted paragraphs.

In doing these Isometric Power Flexes, Swoboda's students became extremely strong, beautifully sculpted, and masters of muscle control. In fact, it was Swoboda who coined the term *muscle control* in 1898 (then featured in his 1901 course) and not Maxick, who began selling his Maxalding course in 1909. Both men used the term *muscle control* to describe the ability to powerfully contract and relax any given muscle group at will.

One other interesting note is that world famous Charles Atlas, perhaps the most famous bodybuilder of all time, was quoted as saying, "Everything I know, I learned from A. P. Swoboda."

Swoboda's books and courses were published by the Roycrofters of East Aurora, New York. They were exquisitely produced at a quality standard that is difficult to find to this very day, and the literary content and knowledge they contained were brilliant.

By 1901, just three years after starting to market "The Swoboda System," Alois P. Swoboda had become a millionaire. The headquarters for his mail-order empire was located in Chicago, Illinois. His course remained until October 1929, when he lost everything in the Stock Market Crash that ushered in the Great Depression of the 1930s. He was working on a comeback when he died in 1939.

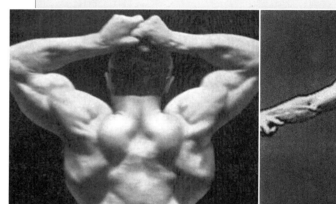
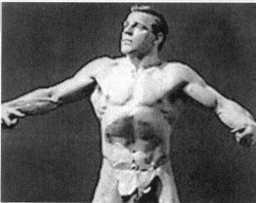
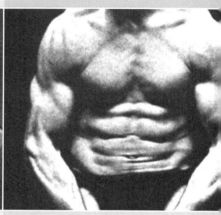

MAXICK

"The Master of Muscle Control"

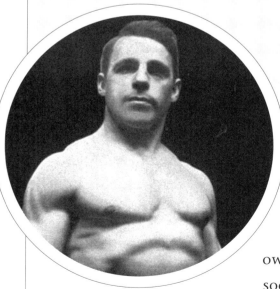

W hile MacFadden and Swoboda were making names for themselves in America in the early 1900s with their own brands of Isometrics and physical culture, there were similar stirrings in Europe. Here there was a young man by the name of Max Sick, who stood less than 5'3" tall but was phenomenally strong and well developed. He was introduced in London, England, by strong man Tromp Van Diggelen, who was a master physical culturist in his own right. Although the two men had never met, they soon discovered that they had both, independently of each other, devised a system of muscle control and physical culture based on Isometric Contraction exercises that allowed them to develop extraordinary robust health as well as great physical strength without the use of any form of apparatus.

It was shades of Alois P. Swoboda and Bernarr MacFadden all over again. In fact, when Van Diggelen met Max Sick, he convinced Max Sick to change his name to "Maxick" in order to appeal to an English audience. (After all, how many English-speaking men would want to purchase a health and muscle building course from a man whose name was Max Sick?) In 1909 this brought into being the world famous "Maxalding" Mail-Order Bodybuilding and physical culture course that remained popular for well over 60 years throughout Europe. Similar to the Swoboda course, which was published in 1898 in America, the Maxalding course featured Isometric Power Flex exercises and made numerous references to directed thought being the source of muscular contraction and the key to the acquisition of great strength.

The following is an excerpt taken from *Muscle Control* by Maxick that was written in 1911 and explains the power of focused thought in achieving success with Maxalding:

How Mechanical Exercise May Hinder Muscle-Development

66 One day I was watching a journey-man filing metal. I fell to wondering vaguely why it was that his arm and deltoid development was so small in comparison with that of the rest of his body, knowing, as I did, that the man had worked at the bench for years. Surely, according to accepted theory, it was just these parts which should be the more developed considering the nature of his work!

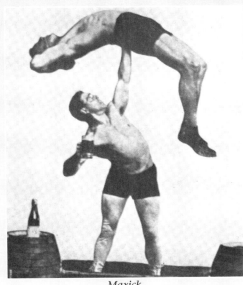

Maxick

I was so interested in this case that I began to take careful note of other workmen; and my observations at length convinced me that *mechanical exercise will not increase bulk of strength beyond a certain degree.*

I found out later by experiment that mechanical exercise will only produce good results if interest is directed to the muscles being used. If the mind is directed only to work being performed, a certain point of muscular resistance is reached; but there it stops. *To secure full benefit from the exercise it is essential that the mind be concentrated on the muscles, and not on the work performed.* 99

The Case of the Stonemason

    " Instances by way of example may be given by the hundred. Take the case of the stonemason, who has to use a hammer or mallet for many hours daily, during which thousands of blows are struck, and the shoulder and arm have to bear the weight, as well as use the mallet.

Now, according to the theories enunciated by many teachers of physical culture, the greater the number of repetitions performed of one exercise, the greater the development of the muscles employed. But here is a flat contradiction of these theories, for it will be observed that the majority of stonemasons do not evince anything exceptional in the way of arm and shoulder muscle development.

And the explanation? Perfectly simple! *The stonemason's mind is necessarily concentrated upon the work before him, and he pays little or no heed to his muscles.* "

Maxick clearly explains why self-directed Isometric Contractions without apparatus can yield such exceptional results. It is because during a true Isometric Contraction, the individual's thoughts or mind is clearly focused on the contraction of the muscle itself.

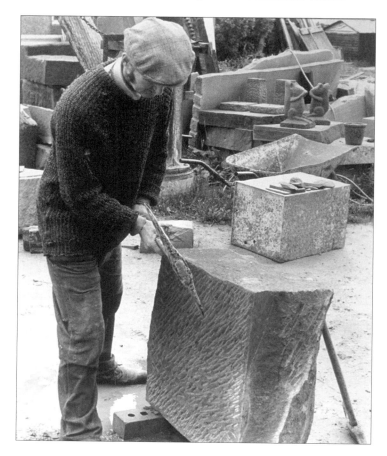

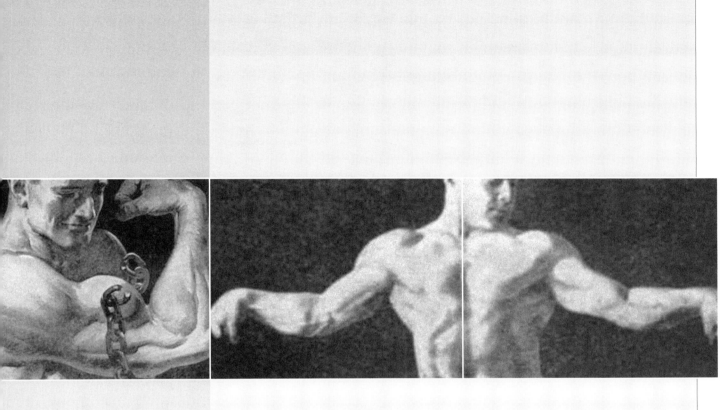

GEORGE F. JOWETT

"Master Physical Culturist, Strongman, and Publisher"

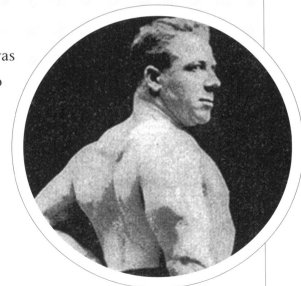

This same concept of mind/muscle connection was also written about by George F. Jowett, who also became famous as a strongman and physical culturist. In his book *The Unrevealed Secrets of Man*, which was published in 1928, Jowett stated the following, which is totally in sync with what Maxick stated in the previous section:

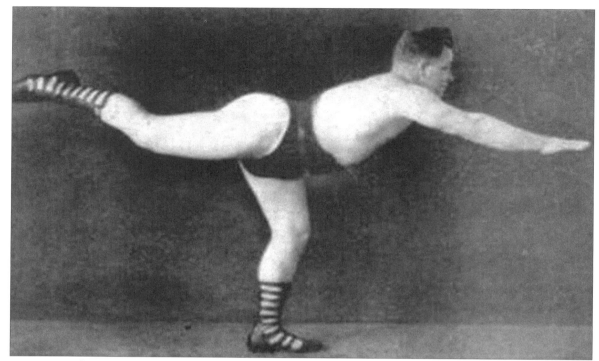

George F. Jowett performing an Isometric balance exercise (try holding that for three minutes!).

❝ Mental concentration is where thousands of bodybuilders fall; they fail to see the dividing line. Blindly they stagger about the road and fail to read the sign at the crossroads. Their case is a reminder of "the spirit is willing but the flesh is weak." You never saw a pitcher successfully curve a ball over the plate while arguing with the umpire. No, and you never saw a body culturist acquire the super state of physical manhood with movements that lacked pep and a mind filled with "Gee whiz, how soon will I be done?" They are like the youngster learning music with his eyes on the clock.

Practicing a movement a hundred times or thousand times will not get you anywhere, nor will pulling and hauling at a ton of iron. *The more mental impulse you put behind an effort the less time is required.* Movements become clockwork, too mechanical, and hauling a ton of metal is like praying to a bronze Buddha to hand you out a check for a million dollars. ❞

As you can clearly see from these quotes taken from Maxick and George F. Jowett, as well as the entire history of Isometric Contraction up to this point, your success with Isometric Contractions as the master method of physical development would seem to be dependent upon two essential factors: (1) The muscular contraction itself and (2) your ability to use your mind and directed thoughts with a laser-like focus to intentionally contract your muscles with great intensity. These two factors are, in fact, two of the golden keys to superior lifelong strength and development. But there is a third equally important factor, literally the third golden key that has been completely overlooked in *all* contemporary Isometric training texts published since the 1950s. And when I say all, I *mean all.* As a result, I can safely say that not one man in a 1,000 is remotely aware of the secret that you are about to learn. To explain the third golden key, I will turn to the writings of the man who introduced Max Sick to the world as Maxick, a man for whom I have tremendous admiration and respect, Tromp Van Diggelen.

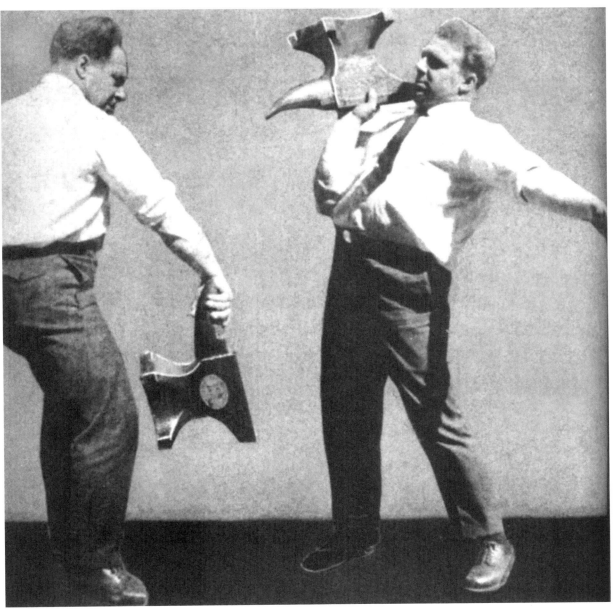

George F. Jowett performing his famous anvil stunt.

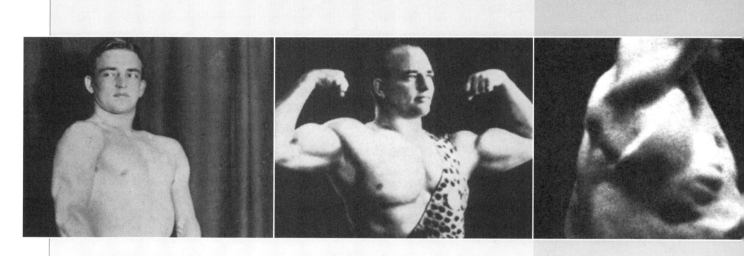

TROMP VAN DIGGELEN

"Adventurer Extraordinaire"

I n his autobiography, titled *Worthwhile Journey,* Tromp Van Diggelen, who was one of the world's greatest physical culturists and one of the world's strongest men, explained his method of (Isometric) muscular contraction and how he discovered it. He also highlighted the *third golden key* that makes Isometric Contraction the superior method that it truly is. Even without employing the third key, you could still achieve tremendous muscular strength and shapeliness, but with it you become master over your entire voluntary muscular system. This key will tremendously enhance your functional strength and athletic ability by having complete muscular control over your entire musculature from the top of your head to your toes. Please read very carefully:

" One day, Mr. Tatham told me that when you pinch a muscle with your fingers you hinder or impede the blood flow in that muscle and then, when the muscle is released, the blood which was kept back, flows forward again with increased impetus. "If you have a little stream of water," he said, "and you hold back the flow by putting a spade across the small furrow, the water builds up behind the spade, and when you lift the spade again, that extra water runs forward strongly." That simple picture made the idea very clear to me, and I responded by saying: "But, Mr. Tatham, if I make the muscle in my arm hard, the blood flow in the muscle must surely be slowed down?" "By Jove, you are right, Cottie," he replied. "Then," I went on, "when I relax the muscle again, the blood must fill it even better than usual for a few moments, and so if I contract my muscles *extra* hard and I relax them again, *extra* well, I will be creating a better blood flow in them, and as you have always told me that the blood is a river of nourishment, I would be bringing extra food to the muscles as well as the nerve-centres, wouldn't I, sir?" "Cottie," said my teacher, "you have said something very important; it seems that it is not

the exercise that develops the muscle but the blood that the exercise brings to the muscles."

We talked the matter over at length, and I told him how I explained to my mother that I was not strong enough to pull rubber strands in an attempt to get stronger. I had told her that I was wasting energy and that I must save the small amount of strength that I possessed.

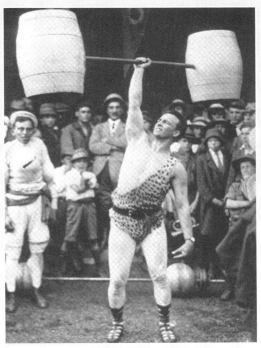

Tromp at a fair in the First World War, lifting 210 pounds with one hand.

Later on, when I had better words at my command, I explained myself more aptly by saying: "One must conserve energy when exercising and *expend* it as little as possible. If, for instance, you swing Indian clubs to develop your pectoral muscles, you will not get the splendid and quick results that you get by strongly contracting these muscles for a couple of seconds, and then relaxing them *thoroughly* for a couple of seconds, and repeating this simple procedure till you feel that the pectoral muscles are properly flushed with blood."

Many, many years later I was very happy when Professor Stibbe, the noted anatomist of the London University, said: "Tromp Van Diggelen is the first man who ever spoke of *forced* relaxation."

As you can see from reading Van Diggelen's text, the third golden key that allows you complete self-mastery over your entire muscular system is your ability to completely *relax* your muscles with the same level of control as that with which you consciously contract them. This allows your circulatory system to bring new nourishment and life-giving oxygen to your muscles, nerves, and every cell of your body. More on Tromp Van Diggelen later, but now I want to introduce you to Alexander Zass, The Amazing Samson.

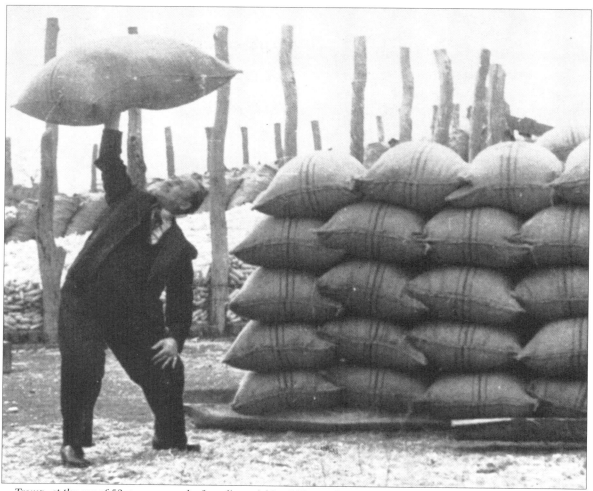

Tromp, at the age of 53, presses a sack of mealies weighing 203 pounds, which was 20 pounds more than his own weight.

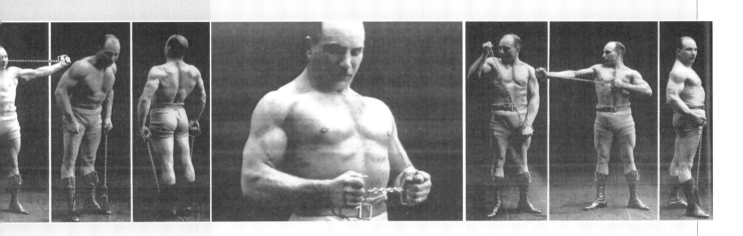

ALEXANDER ZASS

"The Amazing Samson"

O f all the men who have used Isometric Contraction to develop superior strength and physique, I believe that Alexander Zass reigns supreme. At the level of feats of strength for which he was famous, I have no doubt that he truly was the world's strongest man. His claim to fame was his ability to bend thick iron bars and snap chains with his bare hands. But it wasn't just iron bars that Zass could bend. He did, in fact, bend railroad spikes into perfect "U" shapes and did so on several occasions. What made his feats of strength so unique was the way in which he developed his extraordinary strength. That alone is the stuff of legend, and also very reminiscent of what Victor Hugo stated in *Les Misérables* about convicts in prison practicing a "mysterious series of statics" that produced extraordinary strength.

For Alexander Zass, it all started in World War I when he was a Russian prisoner of war in an Austrian prison camp. Prior to the war he had been a very strong man who worked out religiously with conventional training methods of the day and

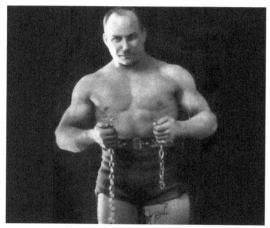
Alexander Zass breaking chains

was very proficient at the art of wrestling. But once imprisoned, he found himself shackled in solitary confinement and unable to exercise properly, or so he thought. Sure enough, his body began to deteriorate just as anyone's body would when it is deprived of exercise. It was then that he began pulling and pushing on his prison bars and chains as a means of exercise. To his great delight, he discovered that not only did this form of training rebuild his strength and physique, but it augmented it far beyond any level that he had enjoyed previously. When the time was right, he bent the bars to his prison

window, ripped one of them out, bent the bar to use as a J-hook for scaling a wall, and literally snapped the chains from his manacles to make good his escape!

After the war, Zass continued with his newly developed strength training method, refined it, went on the road as a strongman throughout Europe and England, and became famous as "The Amazing Samson," performing feats of strength that have not been duplicated to this day. He also sold the very first course that utilizes Isometric Contraction exclusively. In fact, the entire Zass course was conducted using chains as the sole strength building apparatus, just as Zass had used as a prisoner of war. But think about it. What could possibly be more macho than having your students endeavor to break chains? And break chains they did. Several of his best students wrote to him requesting even heavier chains because, like their hero Alexander Zass, they too had broken their chains and needed something more substantial. Such was the power of the Zass Isometric Training method, which was initiated 30 years prior to Isometric Contraction being verified as the superior strength building method by the scientists who conducted hundreds of physical experiments with thousands of test subjects between 1946 and 1961 at the Max Planck Institute in Dortmund, Germany.

I should also mention one other interesting fact. Although Zass was second to none at the feats of strength for which he was famous, he did not possess the right kind of leverage, and therefore strength, to perform heavy feats of weightlifting. In fact, W. A. Pullum, who was the British weightlifting coach in the 1948 Olympic Games, the first Olympics conducted after World War II, spoke in the most complimentary way imaginable about Zass in spite of the fact that Zass was *not* a weightlifter. The following is an excerpt from the October 1952 *Health and Strength* magazine article titled, "Alexander Zass: The Amazing Samson":

"Samson, though, while so popular with the general public, was not so with weightlifters, on the whole, *as he did not do weightlifting in his act.* There were even some who argued that neglect to do this—as he *must* have used weights to gain the strength he possessed—was a betrayal of their favorite sport. Had their anatomical knowledge only been as profound as their convictions, they would have found that far from Samson having manufactured his particular brand of strength with weights, it was evident he had *not* used them in manner understood, the very nature of some of his feats clearly proving that. For these feats had developed to a degree of superhuman strength the muscles *that opposed the actions of orthodox weightlifting.*

Couldn't Do Weightlifting! That's the all-sufficing reason why Samson never featured weightlifting in his act: *he just couldn't do it!* Which further explains why the projected match with Goërner never had the slightest chance of coming off. One was a weightlifting strong man, the other was not. No possibility existed of bringing the two extremes together, or even of effecting a middle course compromise. Samson being in a position where he could dictate terms, naturally could not be expected to compromise."

I have included Pullum's quote to answer a commonly asked question about whether or not Isometric Contraction by itself will make you a better weightlifter. You can see that it will build sheer strength and power better than any other method. But to be good at weightlifting requires speed, excellent leverage, and technique. If you are missing any of these three components, you may be amazingly strong, as was Alexander Zass, and perhaps among the strongest of men worldwide, but not in a way that applies to weightlifting. So instead of using a bar to lift weights, you just bend the bar.

Finally, one more point of interest about Alexander Zass. During the 1920s and 1930s, his course of Chain Isometrics was phenomenally popular in Europe. I can't help but believe that when World War II ended and thousands of injured soldiers desperately needed rehab that the doctors at the Max Planck Institute decided to check out the Zass method only to verify it as the world's best and most efficient method of building muscle strength. More on that later.

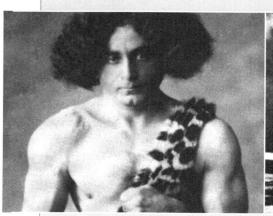 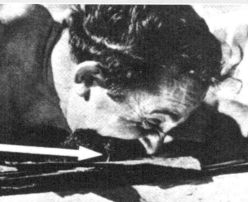 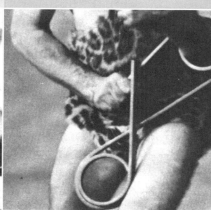

JOSEPH GREENSTEIN
"The Mighty Atom"

At the same time that Alexander Zass was touring the capitals of Europe, performing his magnificent feats of strength to sold-out audiences, there was a Zass-counterpart touring the vaudeville circuit in America and performing many of the same types of feats as Zass. His name was Joseph Greenstein, "The Mighty Atom."

Similar to both Zass and Maxick, Greenstein stood 5'3" tall and weighed 147 pounds. He too was famous for breaking chains, bending bars, and straightening horse-shoes with his bare hands. And similar to Alexander Zass, he trained a great deal with Isometric Contraction. In fact,

Greenstein first learned about Isometric Contraction while accompanying his friend and mentor, the Russian Cossack circus strongman "Volanko," on a trip to India in the summer of 1908. Volanko was visiting his Indian friend, who was known worldwide as the greatest wrestler who ever lived, "Gama, the Lion of the Punjab." The following is an excerpt from the book, *The Mighty Atom: The Life and Times of Joseph L. Greenstein, Biography of a Super Human* by Ed Spielman:

66At last, he and Volanko arrived at a place that was crowded with a chattering throng; they were the only Europeans among them. It was a wrestling ring. For centuries wrestling was the national sport of India, and it was treated with some formality.

In the center of a loose earthen pit, two massive Indian wrestlers stood naked except for breech cloths, their black mustaches preened and heads shaven. Each raised a weighty gold scepter-mace, his badge of championship. This formality concluded, the two men faced each other in the open pit. The crowd took up a chant, calling the name "Gama" again and again as the match began. In a matter of seconds, the smaller man upended his opponent and slammed him to the earth as a roar went up. A gross mismatch. The victor was Volanko's friend, "Gama, the Lion of the Punjab," who would in years to come be recognized by Western sports historians as the

greatest wrestler of the twentieth century.

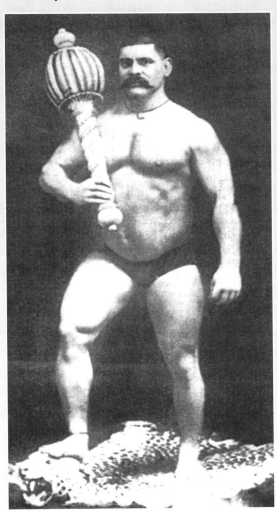

At 5'6" and 270 pounds of solid muscle, The Mighty Gama was undefeated in 5,000 matches. No need to wonder why!

After the match, Volanko, Gama, and the boy sat in the shade as the two wrestlers talked idly and all shared from a large basket of fruit, a gift to Champion Gama who was a strict vegetarian. With appropriate deference, the boy addressed him.

"Gama, may I ask you something?"

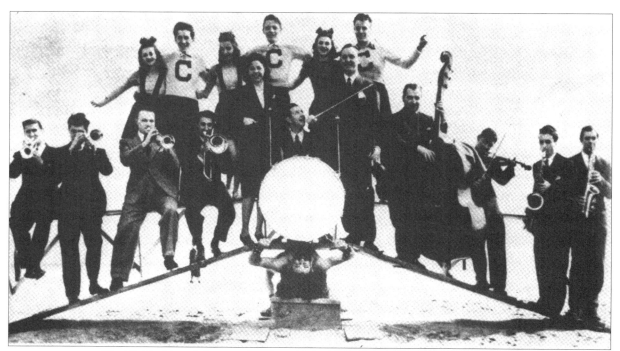

The Mighty Atom, lying on a board studded with sharp-pointed nails, as he supports 17 members of a band and their instruments. He held this position for 15 minutes.

"Ask."

"Your opponent was very big…"

"…and yet I threw him like a baby."

"How?" Yosselle asked in wonderment.

"It's really quite simple," the Indian said good-naturedly. "In the Punjab, where I lived, there was a large tree behind my house. Each morning I would rise up early, tie my belt around it, and try to throw it down."

"A tree?" the boy marveled.

"For twenty years."

"And you did it?"

"No, little one," Gama smiled, "but after a tree…a man is easy." **"**

It was from this introduction to Isometric Contraction that The Mighty Atom began applying the method for the development of his own super human strength. Similar to Alexander Zass, Greenstein was an exceptionally good wrestler and athlete, whose feats amazed onlookers to the point where they literally could not believe what they were seeing. In addition to chain breaking, bar bending, and horseshoe straightening, The Atom also performed a few unorthodox feats. For instance, he would drive a 6" spike through a long 2" X 6" board with a single palm strike. Then he would bend over, use his teeth to extract the spike from the board, and proceed to bite the spike in half. He would also bite through chains as part of his act. Now, I grant you that biting through spikes and chains is extreme and just a little bit strange, but it also demonstrates an unusual level of strength.

The following is an excerpt taken from the June 1938 *Look* magazine in which The Mighty Atom performed the feats I've just mentioned. At the time of the article, The Atom was 55 years old. The fact that his Isometric training method produced exceptional strength is without question. But what is even more amazing was the fact that 38 years later, during the summer of 1976 when he was 93 years old, The Mighty Atom was still performing the same feats of strength! The photographic sequence shown at the bottom of this page was taken at that event more than 30 years ago at Madison Square Garden.

Bottom line: not only will Isometrics make you a great deal stronger, it will help keep you that way for life. And if you do a few other things right, you can expect a very long, healthy, and vigorous life just like The Mighty Atom.

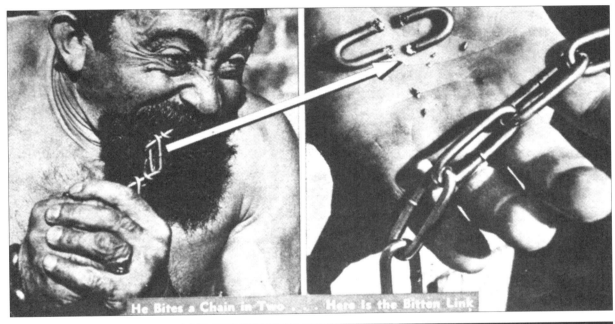

He Bites a Chain in Two . . . . Here Is the Bitten Link

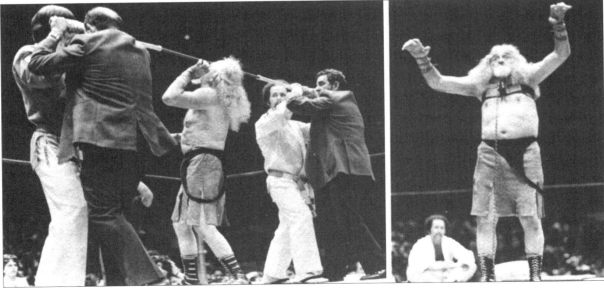

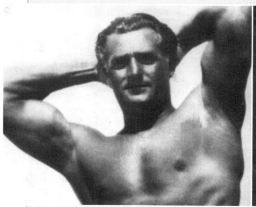 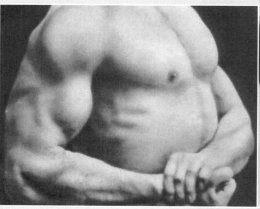 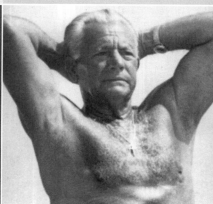

CHARLES ATLAS

"The World's Most Perfectly Developed Man"

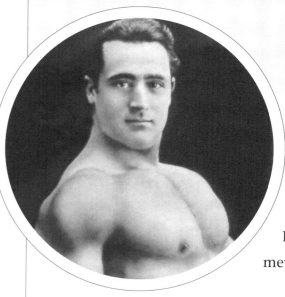

In a very real sense, the history of Isometric Contraction would be totally incomplete and lacking without mention of "The World's Most Perfectly Developed Man," Charles Atlas. It would be like the history of the D-Day invasion of Normandy, France, on June 6, 1944, without the mention of General Dwight D. Eisenhower, the Supreme Commander of the Allied Forces during World War II. After all, when it comes to Isometric Contraction, no one did more to popularize this method of exercise than the legendary Charles Atlas.

So here goes. Charles Atlas was born in Acri, Italy, on October 30, 1893, with the birth name of Angelo Siciliano. He emigrated to the United States with his mother when he was ten years old. During his early teens, he was often victimized by an older bully in a manner nearly identical to the character "Mac" in the famous Charles Atlas cartoon ads— "The Insult That Made a Man Out of Mac"—that were so popular in the comic books of the 1930s–1970s. "Mac" was the skinny guy with the beautiful girl at the beach, and the big bruiser of a bully kicks sand in his face and then threatens to smash in Mac's face. Feeling totally humiliated, Mac sees a "Dynamic Tension" ad in a magazine and writes to Charles Atlas. Within a relatively short period of time, Mac the Scrawny becomes Mac the Mighty, and he looks in the mirror and says, "It didn't take Charles Atlas long to give me these muscles." He then goes back to the same beach, sees the same bully humiliating someone else, and promptly dispatches the idiot with a thunderous right hand and hands the guy's butt to him. Of course, the girl is thrilled and says, "Oh, Mac, you are a real man after all." And there are several other onlookers making statements such as "Wow! Look at that guy's build" and "He's already famous for it."

The truth is that that whole cartoon episode really happened to young Angelo Siciliano. But at the time, he didn't have Charles Atlas to write to, so instead he did the next best thing: he wrote to Alois P. Swoboda. And it was the Swoboda Method that put young Angelo on the fast track to physical transformation and perfection. So much so that one day when Angelo was on the beach with his friends, one of them said, "Hey, Charley [Angelo's nickname], you're looking just like that Atlas guy in the statue." It wasn't long before young Angelo Siciliano legally changed his name to Charles Atlas and became the stuff of legend.

With his newly sculpted physique, Charles Atlas became a highly paid model, posing for many famous sculptors of the day. He also worked at a sideshow on Coney Island, performing as a strongman, and even toured the vaudeville circuit with his friend Earle Liederman in a hand balancing act. Then in 1921, he won the title of "The World's Most Perfectly Developed Man" in a contest sponsored by Bernarr MacFadden and *Physical Culture* magazine. When Atlas won the title again in 1922, MacFadden gave up sponsoring it, saying, "What's the use? Atlas would win it every time."

Atlas then teamed up with Dr. Fredrich Tilney, a noted health writer and physical culturist, and published the world famous Charles Atlas Exercise Course in 1922. Initially, the Atlas course was advertised and promoted primarily in *Physical Culture* magazine and was only moderately successful. But in 1929, Charles Atlas was joined by a young advertising executive by the name of Charles Roman, and they were off to the races. The first thing Roman did was to change the name of the course as well as coin, copyright, and trademark the term for the exercise methods that were featured in the course—"Dynamic Tension." He also rewrote the ads and promotional material so that they appealed as much to teenage boys as to grown men. Hence, there were multiple variations of the ad, "The Insult That Made a Man Out of Mac." Roman ran these ads in comic books, realizing there was an ever-growing army of teens who wanted to become strong and manly like Charles Atlas. In addition, Roman set up

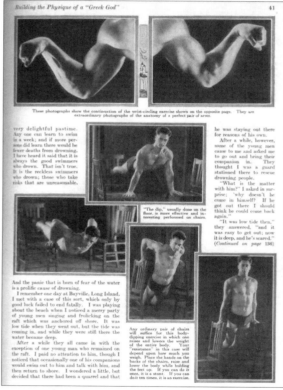

Physical Culture *Magazine*, Dec. 1921

numerous feats of strength for Atlas to perform in public in order to create even more publicity. In fact, throughout the 1930s–1950s, Atlas was never out of the public eye. The team of Altas and Roman was so successful that both men became

millionaires *during* the Great Depression of the 1930s.

It can even further be stated that the Atlas Dynamic Tension Method became the stuff of legend in another way. On February 15, 1933, the superhero "Doc Savage, The Man of Bronze" was introduced in magazine form to an anxious and ever-growing American teen market. (In fact, Lester Dent, who wrote the Doc Savage novels under the pseudonym of Kenneth Robeson, said that his target audience was 15-year-old boys who wanted to become like the superhero Clark "Doc" Savage.) Beginning with the very first issue, Dent made it clear that "Doc" developed his incredible strength and musculature by performing Charles Atlas's Dynamic Tension exercises for two hours every day. And unlike other writers of the day, Lester Dent did not have a weakness for whiskey. According to his wife, when Lester wrote the Savage novels, he was drinking quarts of milk and practicing Dynamic Tension just like the superhero of his novels! That is the type of advertising that money can't buy.

In addition, there were world famous athletes and celebrities of all types who used the Charles Atlas Dynamic Tension exercises. Heavyweight boxing champions Max Baer and Joe Louis, baseball players such as Joe Di Maggio and Ted Williams, and even Robert Ripley proudly stated that he was an Atlas student ("believe it or not"). There was Mahatma Gandhi in far-off India and members of the royal family in Britain, and a future U.S.

president who wrote to Charles Atlas in 1942 in order to become strong enough to pass the enlistment standards for the U.S. Navy. Similar to hundreds of thousands of other young men, John F. Kennedy turned to Charles Atlas in order to get into top physical form and fulfill his patriotic duty by enlisting for World War II, and in the process became a war hero.

After the war, Charles Atlas was a frequent guest on radio programs, and then as television became a media sensation, a whole new generation of America's teenagers was introduced to Charles Atlas and his method of Dynamic Tension. In fact, Mr. Atlas remained popular right up until his death in the early 1970s, and his course is still being sold today by Charles Atlas Limited.

So what exactly is the Charles Atlas Dynamic Tension Method? Simply put, it is a series of dynamic self-resistance exercises for every muscle group in the body that can also be practiced isometrically with no movement at all. These are then

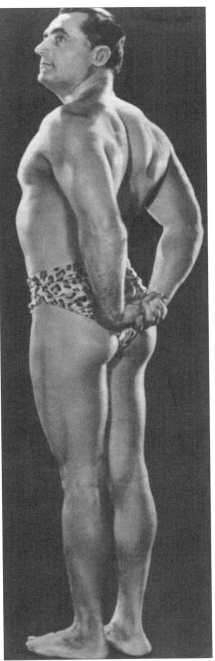

Physical Culture *Magazine, July 1937, age 43*

combined with a selection of power calisthenic exercises for the development of all-around functional strength and fitness. They include many of the same exercises that you find in this book (though we include many more) and yield splendid results. These self-resistance Isometrics can be practiced virtually anytime and anyplace and are the foundation of what my uncle Milo taught me. This form of Isometric Contraction that pits one group of muscles against another is what my uncle Milo termed "Classic Isometric Contraction."

One other interesting piece of information about Charles Atlas and his methods was published in the April 17, 1964 edition of *Life* magazine. The feature article was about the new scientifically verified exercise method called "Isometric Contraction" that had become immensely popular among Americans. Guess what the title was: "Atlas Was Right All Along."

AT LAST! SCIENCE PROVES IT

Although the concept and understanding of Isometric strength training had been known and implemented in various strength building programs around the world for millenniums of time, it had never been scientifically studied, evaluated, validated, or quantified in any way until 1920. And even then, it wasn't studied in the sense of validating or quantifying Isometric strength training. In fact, it was discovered almost completely by accident. And when it was discovered, the results were considered not applicable to human beings and buried in scientific research papers for more than a quarter century.

Here's the scoop on what happened with the first "Isometric Research Project."

The Springfield Study of 1920

In the fall of 1920, a research test was conducted at Springfield College in Springfield, Massachusetts, and the test subjects were frogs. Yes, you read that right: *frogs*. The study was conducted to determine the degenerative effects of immobilization on frogs' legs. The purpose was to observe frogs that had one leg immobilized and the other leg allowed free movement. The idea was to discover how much time was required before the muscles in the immobilized leg would degenerate and atrophy and become virtually nonfunctional.

The context for the experiment is important. It had only been one year since World War I had ended, and there were still thousands of U.S. soldiers in hospitals all around the country who needed rehab before they could return to society. So this test conducted at Springfield College on frogs could be useful in determining how long before complete immobilization caused excessive muscle degeneration and atrophy in humans...or so they thought.

The researchers took healthy frogs and tethered one leg so that it was completely immobile while the other leg was allowed free movement. The results were totally unexpected. After the frogs had been tethered for two weeks, and the tethered leg was released from its harness, the scientists were shocked to discover that the frogs *increased* strength in *the tethered immobilized leg* to an extraordinary degree. So much so that each frog jumped lopsided, because of the incredible strength increase in the tethered leg. After several additional experiments were conducted, with each experiment achieving the exact same result, the research project was abandoned because it seemed there was no application to human beings. The research was written up in scientific journals of the day, but for all intents and purposes was completely disregarded as irrelevant to human beings.

In short, the researchers conducting the experiment at Springfield College were unable to grasp the fact that the reason for the tremendous strength increase in the tethered leg as opposed to the free leg was because the frogs were only using a small precentage of their muscle fibers to move the free untethered leg.

In the immobolized leg, however, by straining against an immovable bond, the entire muscle was exercised to its very deepest muscle fibers. Hence the phenomenal increase in the strength of the tethered leg.

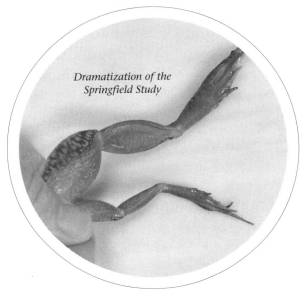

Dramatization of the Springfield Study

As it turned out, the researchers simply did not grasp that they had made an incredible discovery that could have made a huge difference in rehabbing the soldiers from World War I. They simply didn't "get it," and the results of the experiment were shelved until…

1946

It has been said that "necessity is the mother of invention," and that was absolutely true at the end of World War II in 1946. Europe, and particularly Germany, had literally been devastated and destroyed by the carnage of the war, and there was the tremendous *necessity* to rebuild the European continent. Even more acutely felt was the need to rehabilitate tens of thousands of severely injured European soldiers from all sides, both Axis and Allies. By the war's end, there were so many wounded and crippled people that there was not enough medical personnel, medical supplies, hospital beds, or conventional equipment available for rehabilitation. There was a great necessity to return these men to productive civilian enterprise in order to begin the process of rebuilding Europe, but no way to achieve it.

It was then that doctors and physiologists under the direction of Dr. E. A. Müeller and Dr. Theodore Hettinger at the Max Planck Institute in Dortmund, Germany, began an earnest study of Isometric Contraction. The purpose of their study was to determine whether or not Isometric Contraction could be successfully used therapeutically in the rehabilitation of the thousands of injured soldiers who were being returned to civilian life.

At this point, you may wonder why Drs. Müeller and Hettinger chose to specifically focus on Isometric Contraction. I'm not sure that anyone knows the complete answer, but I'll venture a hunch based on the previous history we've already established. By 1946, the Maxalding method of strength and bodybuilding, which was a series of deep Isometric muscle contractions followed by complete relaxation of any given muscle group (hence *muscle control* in both contraction and relaxation), had been made widely popular throughout Europe for more than 35 years. Similarly, Alexander Zass,

"The Amazing Samson," had performed as a strongman to sold-out audiences in virtually all the European capitals throughout all of the 1920s and most of the 1930s. His mail-order bodybuilding course was made up almost exclusively of Isometric strength building techniques, and his method was widely advertised in physical culture journals throughout Europe. Then, of course, by the mid 1930s, Charles Atlas had become internationally famous and was selling his course all over the world, including all of Europe.

So, in retrospect, I have no doubt that faced with the dilemma of tens of thousands of injured soldiers in desperate need of rehabilitation as well as the fact that medical supplies and personnel were grossly inadequate to meet the demand, the researchers at the Max Planck Institute were probably wondering whether or not these strength training methods they had heard about since their youth were in fact *real*; and if they were real, how long before the results were substantive. It was these questions that the researchers at the Max Planck Institute set out to answer, and answer them they did!

In fact, they left no stone uncovered in determining exactly what variables created the best possible results as regards Isometric Contraction. Everything from intensity of contraction (how close to its absolute limit did a muscle have to be contracted in order to obtain the best possible result), time under contraction (its duration), number of contractions required at any given time, and the frequency of contraction in order to obtain the best possible results. These variables were tested and retested on more than 5,000 volunteer test subjects and carefully quantified. The researchers also included other variables besides Isometric Contraction, including nutrition, exposure to ultraviolet light (sunlight), ambient temperature, sleep habits, recreation, and chronological age.

All in all, it was the most extensive research into the physiology of exercise that had ever been conducted up to that point in time. And the results, compiled from experiments lasting more than a decade, are valid to this day.

For instance, going back to the 1920 Springfield Frog Experiment, the researchers at Max Planck conducted much the same experiment but used human test subjects instead of frogs. This is how it was done. A test group comprised of 50 healthy men, ages 19–55, was selected. The strength of each man's arms was carefully measured, then one arm was placed in a plaster cast (okay, so they didn't tether it). This arm received no exercise at all, except *once a day* when the cast was opened and the subjects performed a series of three Isometric contractions for both flexors and extensors of the arm. This arm received a total time expenditure of *less than one minute of exercise a day*. At the end of four weeks, new tests were conducted to determine the results. Of course, there were many variations made to this one basic study, but they all added up to the same results: *dramatic strength increase in the immobolized arm!*

Time after time the results verified themselves, and Isometric Contraction became widely used and endorsed by the medical establishment worldwide as the best, safest, most efficient, and least expensive method of physical rehabilitation of its day. This was also true here in America, where it was being used in the rehabilitation of polio victims.

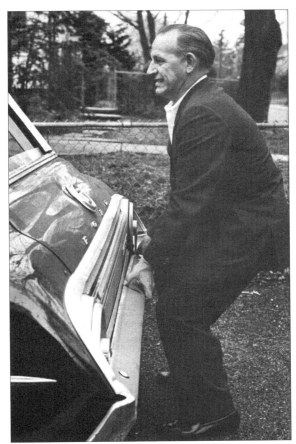

Vic Obeck performing an Isometric Contraction

For example, one of America's preeminent Isometric researchers was Victor Obeck, Professor of Physical Education as well as Director of Athletics at New York University. He had been a professional football player as well as a great all-around athlete prior to his career in academia. Bottom line: he knew a great deal about exercise. But it wasn't until 1960 that he was introduced to Isometric Contraction. It happened during a technical meeting at the Institute of Human Anatomy at the University of Rome during the 1960 Olympic games. There he met a young researcher from the Max Planck Institute who described experiments on the Isometric Contraction of muscles that his director, Dr. E. A. Müeller, had carried out on more than 5,000 volunteers over a period of well over a decade. The results, the young man said, were nothing less than extraordinary.

It was then that Obeck decided to perform his own research into the science of Isometric Contraction. Before long, he was completely convinced and began devising Isometric programs for his athletic teams at New York University and did so with great success. He also stated the following about the therapeutic advantage of Isometric Contraction in his book *Isometrics: How to Exercise Without Moving a Muscle.*

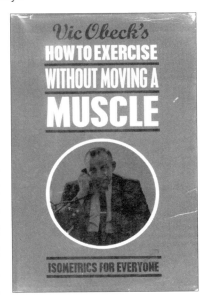

❝One of our students at N.Y.U. had suffered an attack of polio which left his left leg seriously weakened. He'd been trying to build up the lost strength by exercising with weights strapped to his foot. When I first saw him, he could lift a 3-pound weight three times with his weakened leg, 10 pounds ten times with the right one. I suggested he try Isometric exercises for his left leg, while continuing the weights with his right leg. At the end of one month, he could lift a 15-pound weight ten times with his "weak" leg. With the sound leg he could only lift 11 pounds ten times!"

The reason I note this point is because back during the mid 1960s, my uncle Milo purchased Obeck's book and made a point of contacting him. In fact, the two become fairly good friends, and the one thing Obeck came to believe was that the "average" results achieved by volunteer test subjects at the Max Planck Institute *could be greatly surpassed by motivated individuals.*

And what were the averages according to the researchers at the Max Planck Institute? Well, the truth is that it varied with the individual and the various muscle groups. The following excerpt is from Dr. Theodore Hettinger's book, *The Physiology of Strength,* which was first published in America in 1961. The paragraph cited and the chart are from page 38 and refer to one individual's results. As you can see, the percentage of weekly increase varies by muscle group considerably. And as you can also clearly see, Hettinger stated that the results in the accompanying chart were only representative of that specific individual.

"In Figure 7, as an example, the results of increasing strength during a period of training are given on one

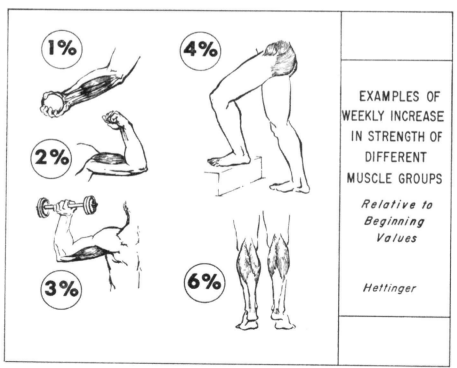

Figure 7

person in whom we have trained many different muscle groups. The numbers demonstrate the increase in strength week by week in percentage of the beginning value. The speed of increase in the different muscle groups is true in these given numbers only for this subject." 99

The point is that although most Isometric Contraction researchers agreed that *weekly increases in strength averaged about 5 percent per week,* there certainly were exceptions. Obeck's student who went from 3 repetitions with 3 pounds to 10 repetitions with 15 pounds in the course of one month using Isometric training alone had an increase in his *functional* strength of 500 percent and a simultaneous increase in muscular endurance of more than 300 percent. This was obviously exceptional, and the young man who achieved these results was highly motivated. Thus, based on his own studies, Obeck believed it was possible to greatly surpass the *average* strength increases of the Max Planck research subjects and to even double strength within a relatively short period of time.

This was also verified by another Isometric researcher, Professor James A. Baley of the University of Connecticut. Baley agreed wholeheartedly with Obeck and stated his observations on several occasions. In his *Illustrated Guide to Developing Athletic Strength, Power, and Agility,* Baley stated, "The same results can be achieved in a twenty-five minute session with Isometrics as can in a two-hour session with barbells." In fact, when Professor Baley put Isometrics to the test with a class of college students at the University of Connecticut, the Isometric training group improved *three times faster* than the sports training group on tests measuring increases in strength, *endurance,* coordination, and agility.

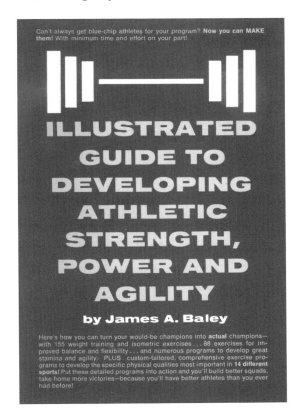

I especially like to shine a spotlight on the *increased endurance* benefits of Isometrics that both Obeck and Baley verified. Why? Because one of the biggest myths perpetuated about Isometric training is that it will not increase *endurance.* That assertion is absolutely false. Isometrics, when properly applied, can and will build phenomenal muscular endurance. Obeck's student, who was mentioned previously, is a perfect example.

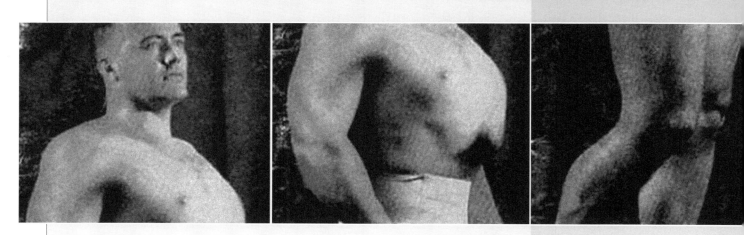

BOB HOFFMAN

Captain America and the "Cold War"

Although the heyday of Isometric training in the U.S. was from 1960 to 1968, it had actually been used by the American Olympic Weightlifting Team soon after 1954 with spectacular results. At the time, Bob Hoffman, founder of The York Barbell Company in York, Pennsylvania, was the coach of the Olympic team. During that Cold War era, the Soviets were dominating in weightlifting at both the Olympics and the World Championships, which Hoffman regarded with sheer contempt. Bob Hoffman was known as the world's most patriotic egomaniac, a totally self-made man who worshiped his creator and as a man who hated to lose, and it showed!

He so hated to lose that he was willing to do *anything* to win, especially to beat the Soviets. In fact, if he had had his way, America would have nuked the Soviet Union during the Soviet Missile Crisis in 1962! But back in the 1950s, the only way Hoffman could have his victory over the Soviets was in the arena of weightlifting. When his U.S. team had their "butts handed to them" by the Soviets in 1954, Hoffman was furious. He immediately enlisted his friend, Dr. John Ziegler, who was the physician to the U.S. Olympic Weightlifting Team, to find out how it was possible that the Soviets had so humiliated the Americans. It wasn't long before Ziegler had the answers. It came down to two factors. First, the Soviets were using a new training method that German doctors had developed called "Isometrics." And, second, the Soviets were using synthetic derivatives of testosterone with which they were injecting their weightlifters. Bottom line: the Soviets were using steroids.

As soon as Hoffman found out, he didn't blow the whistle on the Soviets for doping. Instead, he had Dr. Ziegler work with CIBA Pharmaceuticals to develop far better steroids than anything the Soviets were taking and to also use the Isometric training techniques that the Soviets were using to train his American athletes. Sure enough, the results were extraordinary, and it wasn't long before Hoffman's U.S. teams were beating the Soviets. But, being the shrewd man who he was, Hoffman kept everything hidden. He even had Dr. Ziegler tell his lifters that they were receiving Vitamin B12 shots so they would not resist taking steroids for fear of long-term health consequences that were unknown in 1954.

As far as Hoffman being afraid of a drug scandal back in the late 1950s and early 1960s, he wasn't. His reasoning was actually quite logical: "What are they [the Soviets] gonna do, tell the judges that our guys are using better dope than theirs?" Still, Hoffman wasn't about to tell the American public that our weightlifters were using steroids, so he told a half truth—our guys were using a new strength training method called "Functional Isometric Contraction," in order to shatter the existing weightlifting records of the day.

One other thing about Bob Hoffman. Those who knew him said he was "basically an honest guy." Hearing that, my grandfather's friend, Uncle Wally, used to say,

"WHEN A MAN SAYS HE'S *basically honest, that means* **HE ONLY LIES WHEN HE NEEDS TO."**

THE ISOMETRIC BOOM OF THE 1960S

By the 1960s, Isometrics had became a phenomenally popular method of strength building for athletes in all sports, moving well beyond the weightlifting crowd. In fact, in 1961, Mickey Mantle and Roger Maris, who were roommates when the New York Yankees were on the road, were

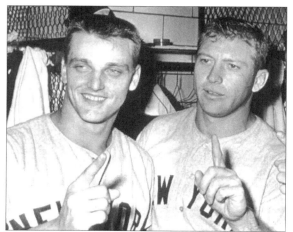

Roger Maris (left) and Mickey Mantle

both using Isometrics during their famous home run derby. Ultimately, Maris won with a grand total of 61 and became the first man to eclipse Babe Ruth's record of 60 home runs that had been set in 1927. Oddly enough, when the endorsers were looking for a baseball star to endorse a new Isometric exerciser, they turned to Mickey Mantle rather than Roger Maris. Why? Because the public loved Mantle, and the Mick was the man whom the public wanted to be the first to top Babe Ruth's record. When that didn't happen, many fans actually turned against Roger Maris.

But in addition to Mickey Mantle, there were also other athletes and celebrities who endorsed Isometric exercises. Even President Kennedy practiced Isometrics on a daily basis on the advice of the White House physician. To Kennedy, it was nothing new. He was just resuming the Charles Atlas exercises that he had used some 20 years previous.

By 1964, the Isometric rage was in full swing in America, and there were books and magazines on newsstands everywhere with idiotic titles, such as *Isometrics: Total Fitness Without Effort, The Lazy Man's Guide to Physical Fitness,* and many, many more. While some books were better than others, many were written by people who obviously didn't know a true Isometric Contraction from a hole in the ground. Hence, the ridiculous titles.

This brings up a point I want to reiterate. The words *easy* and *Isometric Contraction* should never be used in the same sentence unless the person is saying that Isometric exercises are *easy* to learn. That part may be true. BUT *no way are they easy to do!* Just the opposite is true. Isometrics are not even remotely easy to do. They require a laser-like focus with deep concentration and require that you exert yourself from 7 to 12 seconds at roughly two-thirds of your maximum strength. Of course, there are other Isometric protocols that are shorter in duration, such as 1 to 2 seconds at 95 to 100 percent of one's strength, but doing so could also put one at risk of severe injury. So those *are not recommended* in this book as practical for our purposes. Another Isometric protocol is what has been coined "Aerobic Isometrics" by strongman Steve Justa, a man for whom I have great respect. Mr. Justa recommends Isometrics of all durations and intensities with some performed at 35 percent of perceived maximum strength and held for 30 seconds to several minutes. This is what he refers to as "Aerobic" Isometrics, and trust me, those are tough. More on Steve Justa to come.

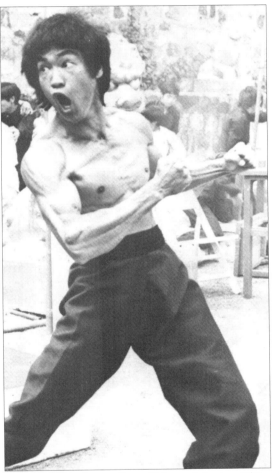
Bruce Lee, on the set of one of his martial arts movies

Isometrics were used to great effect by a wide range of people from all walks of life during the 1960s. They were even used by some doctors to treat hypertension successfully. One celebrity who turned to Isometrics was the late Bruce Lee of martial arts fame. Lee had injured his back so severely in a weight training accident that he never lived another day without agonizing pain. (It's been substantiated that prescription painkillers were implicated in his death.) After the accident, Bruce Lee became an Isometric fanatic and experimented with every variable of intensity and duration imaginable. The result was a "ripped to the bone" muscularity that was incredible to behold, even though he did not have great muscular size. At 5'7", Mr. Lee weighed less than 140 pounds. Nonetheless, Chuck Norris, the martial artist and movie/TV star, said that Bruce Lee was the strongest man of his size whom he had ever met. And the reason for it? Isometrics!

So what kind of Isometrics did Bruce Lee perform? That's where Steve Justa comes in. In his masterful book, *Rock, Iron, Steel*, which was published in 1998, Justa recounted one Isometric technique that Bruce Lee sometimes practiced that I had never read about. Here's how it's done. Take a 3-pound steel ball and hold it in your palm with your arm straight out in front of you and fingers pointing down. As soon as your arm tires, switch to the other arm in exactly the same position while allowing the tired arm to rest. Continue to switch back and forth. Sounds easy enough, right? Anyone can do it, right? Okay, now here's the kicker. Do it for 8 hours straight without a break. Seriously, that's exactly what Bruce Lee did.

What do you suppose the results of such an extreme Isometric exercise would be? Even with a weight that light, over the course of time the entire body would come into play. You'd literally be pulling from your toes to the top of your head, and after 8 hours the effect it would give your whole body—and I mean your *whole* body—would be that it would feel like a steel cable, like it is one unit of rock-hard strength and muscle. But even if you wanted to duplicate such an extreme endeavor, who has that much time? This is where Steve Justa came up with his concept of Aerobic Isometrics, where one uses a perceived 35 percent of maximum contraction and holds it for periods of up to 3 minutes or even longer if you're fanatical

about it. Even though 35 percent may not sound all that intense, I assure you from personal experience that as the muscle fibers begin fatiguing and new ones are recruited, it isn't long before even the very deepest muscle fibers are engaged. And the result? Well, several members of the Bronze Bow forum have applied these same techniques of Aerobic Isometrics to pull-ups and other exercises, and to a man they all agree with me that their muscular strength, definition, and endurance go through the roof.

But perhaps best of all is the *carryover* to everyday, real world functional strength that these exercises will enhance to a tremendous extent. To make the point perfectly, let me give you another example

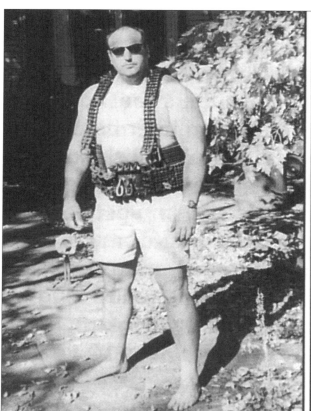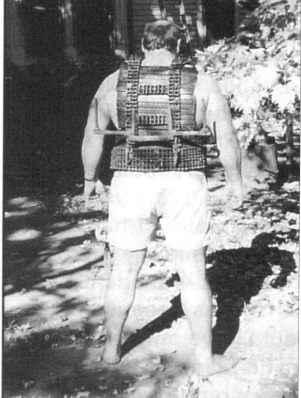

Steve Justa modeling his one of a kind weight vest

from Steve Justa's book, where he devotes an entire chapter to Isometrics. According to Justa, an avid strength trainee who lifts tremendous weights as well as odd objects such as 450-pound barrels, Isometrics gave him functional strength that he simply could not acquire from weightlifting. He tells the story about baling hay for a man who was half his size and had Bruce Lee type of muscular definition, but who was at least twice as strong as Justa in this form of manual labor. Justa desperately wanted to keep up with this man,

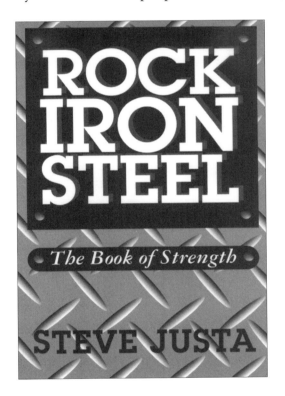

and despite two years of the most intense and brutal heavy weight training imaginable, in which his weightlifting strength doubled, Justa was shocked to discover that he was no stronger in baling hay than when he started. Quite literally, although he could lift weights that were twice as heavy, there was little if any carryover.

Then something clicked. He remembered Bruce Lee and Isometrics. So instead of lifting weights, he pushed, pulled, and pried against an immovable object with no weight training at all for 3 months. He tried widely varied intensities and durations. And the result? Within 3 months his hay baling strength had improved by 40 percent. So think it through. No improvement in 2 years on the heavy weights. Forty percent better within 3 months of Isometrics. That, to me, my friends, is one of the primary benefits of Isometric strength training and muscle sculpting. Simply put, Isometrics make you functionally stronger in a way that nothing else can. And when your muscles become so much stronger in a functional sense as a result of Isometric training, you'll start experiencing what so many of my students have stated—your body will feel so much lighter and you will have greater endurance. Why? Because when you double your strength with Isometrics, your body will feel half as heavy, and you'll find that you move with greater economy and a new spring in your step.

This brings us to the next major benefit of Isometric Contraction for strength building. And what might that be? How does Perpetual Youth sound?

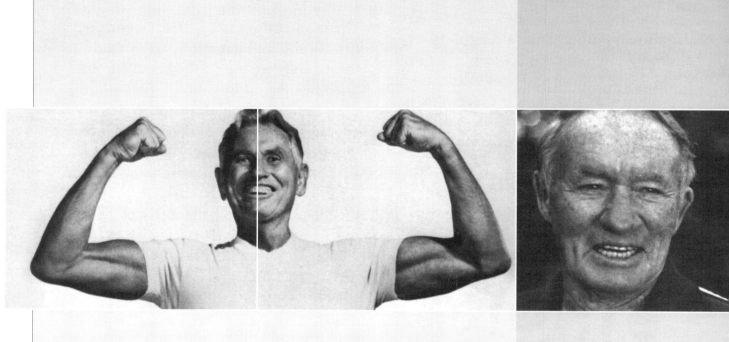

PAUL BRAGG & NOEL JOHNSON
Proof That Growin' Old Ain't for Sissies!

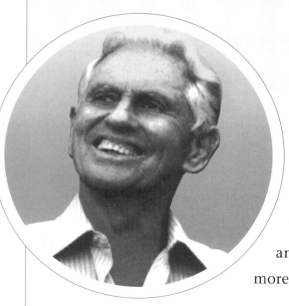

PAUL BRAGG'S BUILT TO LAST FORMULA FOR ETERNAL YOUTH

Throughout the 1960s and into the mid 1970s, a physical culturist by the name of Paul Bragg was becoming something of a cult figure. At the time of his premature death due to a surfing accident in 1976, Bragg was 95 years old and considered by many to be the personification of everything he taught. Handsome and muscular, Bragg was a prolific author, having written more than 20 books on all facets of physical culture.

If you've read Bragg's books, you know that he wrote with the voice of experience. In fact, as a young teen he had nearly died of tuberculosis, but through a program of carefully applied physical culture he was not only completely made well but was a beautifully sculpted young athlete by the time he turned 20 in 1901. He became a physical culture writer and researcher for Bernarr MacFadden's *Physical Culture* magazine.

As a magazine correspondent, Bragg traveled the entire world in Indiana Jones' fashion. But rather than search for the Lost Ark of the Covenant, Bragg was looking for the secrets—the real secrets—of perpetual strength and youthfulness. And slowly but surely, piece by piece, he discovered the answers during his worldwide travels and wrote and lectured about them. Eventually, he became one of the most widely regarded physical culturists,

with a following that included Jack La Lanne (who credits Bragg with saving his life), Olympic athletes, movie stars, as well as people from all walks of life.

So what exactly was Bragg's perpetual youth formula?

First, he taught deep breathing (just as I teach in this book) as the preeminent requirement for lifelong strength and youthfulness. In fact, he was quick to point out that deep breathing more than anything else was responsible for his return to health and becoming the personification of manly strength and fitness.

He also taught the importance of holistic natural nutrition. And though he was criticized by some for not being a strict vegetarian, he was quick to point out that the healthiest and most long-lived people whom he had met in his worldwide travels

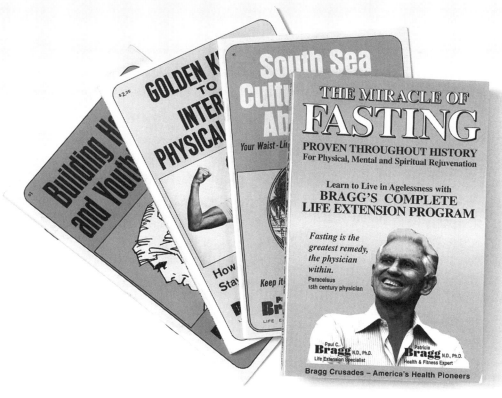

were not strict vegetarians. When challenged even further, he noted that humans have pepsin in their stomachs, which both carnivorous and omnivorous animals in the wild have, but vegetarian animals do not. The bottom line was that this man was so knowledgeable that there was no way that anyone was going to win an argument with him. Bragg even wrote a book titled, *The Shocking Truth About Water,* in which he detailed everything we now know about the importance of pure fresh water for health and longevity. That was more than 40 years ago!

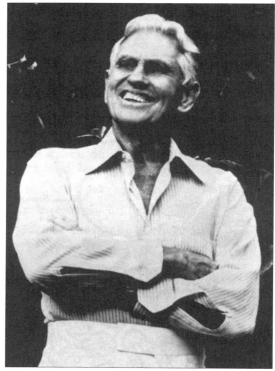

Slim and muscular Paul Bragg at the age of 92

As far as exercise goes, Bragg taught a series of calisthenic exercises for every muscle group as well as Isometrics, which he taught as the ultimate form of strength building exercise in his book, *Building Health and Youthfulness*. Simply put, Paul

Bragg was light years ahead of his time, just as Swoboda and MacFadden had been. Had it not been his premature death in 1975 at the age of 95, one can only wonder how long he would have lived. He might still be surfing.

Was he really in that excellent of shape? When Bragg was introduced as a guest on the *Merv Griffin* television show shortly before his death, the first thing he did was challenge Merv to "Go ahead and hit me in the abdomen as hard as you can. But be careful to not break your wrist." From then on Bragg had the crowd eating out of his hand.

On a final note, when interviewed by *People* magazine when he as 94 years old, Bragg was asked at what age a man loses his sexual desire for beautiful women. The writer of the article said that Bragg looked him right in the eye and said, "You'll have to ask somebody else that question. I'm only 94." And then he winked.

NOEL JOHNSON—A DUD AT 70, A STUD AT 80

In August 1979, my friend Linda Wilkinson introduced me to a remarkable man. His name was Noel Johnson, and he was 80 years old—or should I say 80 years young? At the time, Noel had recently won a gold medal for boxing in the Senior Olympics, having decked a 40-year-old man on the way to the title, and he was looking forward to running in the New York City Marathon in October of that year. To say that Noel was extraordinary would be an understatement. In truth, his story was extraordinary in many ways.

Noel was born on July 7, 1899, in Heron Lake, Minnesota. He grew up on a farm and was strong and healthy as a youngster. When he was in his mid teens, he ordered the mail-order correspondence course from Farmer Burns, "Lessons in Wrestling and Physical Culture," and became an excellent wrestler. A few years later, he ordered the famous Earle Liederman Muscle Building Course.

Although he enjoyed wrestling, Noel soon discovered he had a natural talent for boxing and was able to parlay his physical gifts into a promising career as a professional lightweight boxer. His only serious problem was that as he knocked out one opponent after another, it became harder and harder to find opponents close to home who were willing to get in the ring with him. Not only that, but the managers of other fighters were absolutely adamant about keeping their fighters away from him for fear he would knock them out. Promoters took note of him and before long were warning to watch out for "Battlin' Blue Eyes." So that meant he had to travel farther from home in order to find promoters and managers who didn't know who he was.

Noel fought until age 33, leaving the ring in 1932 to take a job with Texaco Oil in California and focus on raising a family. It wasn't long before he and his family were living the typical American lifestyle, and not long before he started packing on the pounds and losing his beautifully chiseled physique. But he was realizing the American dream, right? That included too much food, too little exercise, too many cigarettes, and too much alcohol.

As the years zoomed by, Noel developed a mild heart condition that became worse and worse along with the accompanying high blood pressure, gout, arthritis, bursitis, hemorrhoids, and a host of other chronic diseases. He told me he was taking so many medications that he finally asked his doctor, "What's the blue pill for?" The doctor said it was there to remind him to take all the others. Worse yet, when he finally reached retirement age, all the things he intended to do and all the places he intended to go with his beloved wife, Zola, were no longer possible. Why? Read this short excerpt from Noel's book, *A Dud at 70, a Stud at 80.*

*Noel Johnson
at the age of 90*

66When I went to work for Convair in 1939, I weighed 130 pounds and was in relatively good health. Looking back now and with the advantage of hindsight, I expect my body began to really deteriorate about the time I stopped fighting professionally. There was no longer the urgency to keep in shape, and our lifestyle, the average American "good life," included smoking, eating anything and everything I wanted, and a lot of social drinking. When I retired in 1964, 25 years later, I weighed 170 pounds and was in bad physical condition.

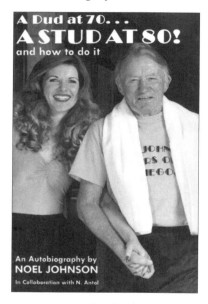

The result was inevitable. There is just no way you or I or anyone else can ignore the basic laws of nature and not wind up in the same shape I found myself in at age 65. Lack of exercise, coupled with nutritionally empty dead food, alcohol, and tobacco, made me a complete dud. Although Zola and I had many interesting things we really wanted to do after I retired, we never got to do any of them. Neither one of us had the energy or the get-up-and-go to leave the house and enjoy our plans. Out of the main-stream of life, we were retired from everything.**"**

Perhaps you're wondering, *C'mon, John, what does this have to do with Isometrics?* Well, I'll tell you what, just hang tight and I'll get to that. I am sharing Noel's story with you because I want to motivate you to take your life, all facets of your life, very seriously. I assure you that if you do nothing to take charge of your health and fitness, you'll end up just like Noel. Now back to his story.

Shortly after Noel's retirement began, his wife, Zola, had a series of strokes, and by the time he was 70, Noel was alone. But still something stirred in him, and he wasn't about to give up on life or love. This is how he describes what happened next in his book (page 59).

"I finally did something I had been carefully avoiding for a long time. I thought. I used the intelligence the Creator had given me. My mind was as rusty and unused as my body, but I persisted and gradually ideas began to form.

I was very clear on what I *didn't* want. I didn't want to be a burden to my children. I didn't want to be bed-ridden and helpless. I felt it was still my personal responsibility to take charge of my own life and health, and I didn't want to turn that responsibility over to anyone else.

First, I stripped down and looked in the mirror. All the classic signs of aging and ill-health were there. I was overweight, with a bulging gut, lack-luster eyes, with unused muscles hanging slack. I looked defeated. But I used to be a fighter, and the thought "defeated" stirred something in my ego. Here I was, about to give up and take the count. I decided then and there to beat the bell and come out swinging. They can't count you out when you're trying.**"**

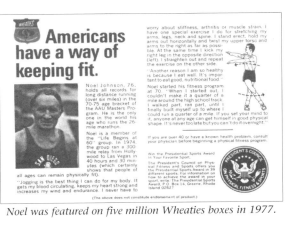

Noel was featured on five million Wheaties boxes in 1977.

"BATTLIN' BLUE EYES" MAKES A COMEBACK!

Immediately after making his decision to "come out swinging," Noel took action. He went to the World of Health food store and talked with a knowledgeable woman about his present condition and told her what he intended to do about it. When he asked her if she had any recommendations, she said, "Follow me." When they got to the book section of the store, she pointed to a series of books that she said were exactly what he needed. They were the "Physical Culture" library of Paul Bragg.

Noel told me that he tore into the Bragg books and couldn't get enough. Everything Bragg said made perfect sense. He started eating right, exercising right, and before long every debilitating health condition he had experienced over the past 40 years vanished—totally disappeared. So much so that in 1971, at the age of 73, newspapers all over California were running articles about him with titles such as "Superman Is Studied at UCD" (University of California at Davis). The articles emphasized that he had won three gold medals in the Senior Olympics that year—for the marathon (26

miles, 385 yards), the mile, and the 10,000-meter races.

From there, Noel decided he wanted to resume boxing. But in order to do that, he needed to dramatically increase his punching strength and power. So he contacted Paul Bragg in Hawaii and arranged to pay him a visit. When Noel met Bragg in 1973, he said he could hardly believe it. Here was a 92-year-old man (18 years Noel's senior) who was the personification of strength, fitness, and vibrant energy! As they talked, Noel asked Bragg what he would recommend to give himself "an edge" in boxing. Without missing a beat, Bragg told him *Isometrics*. And Bragg actually showed him the right selection of Isometric exercises to maximize his punching power.

The rest is history. Noel went on to win and defend his boxing title year after year and was a champion all the way. His radio interviews and television appearances were the stuff of legends, and he was even featured on five million Wheaties Breakfast of Champions boxes that profiled his extraordinary exploits.

When Noel went to be with the Lord in 1995 at the age of 96, one thing is certain: after turning his life around at the age of 70, Noel Johnson was living proof for more than 25 years, as had been his friend Paul Bragg, that "growin' old ain't for sissies."

Well, that's it for the History of Isometrics. There are many scientific papers that I could have referenced, but the way I see it, if you're not convinced by now, you never will be.

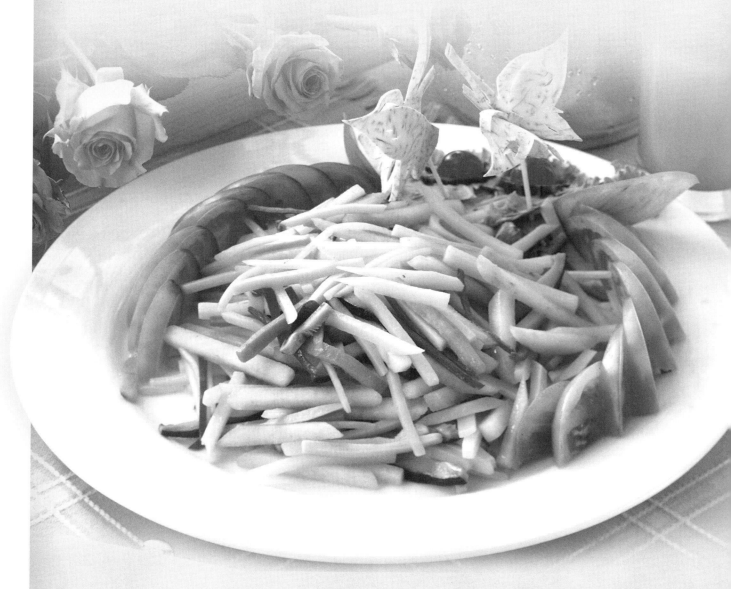

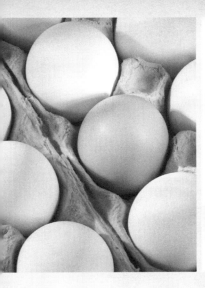
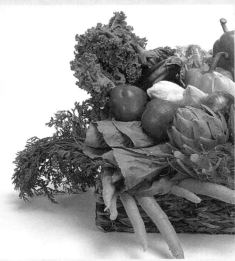
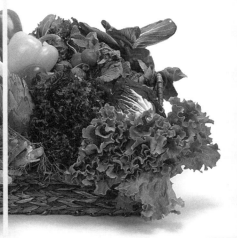

NUTRITION *for* HEALTH, STRENGTH, & LIFELONG VITALITY

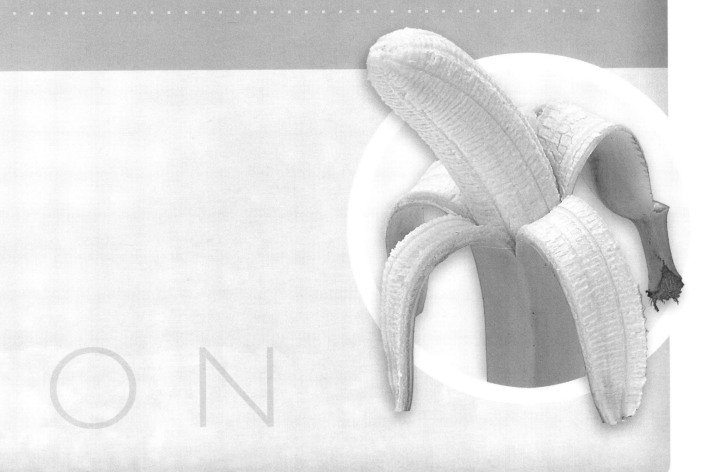

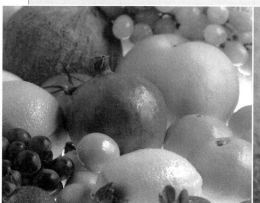
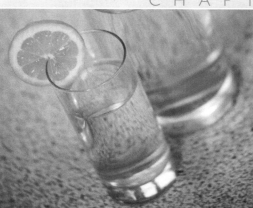
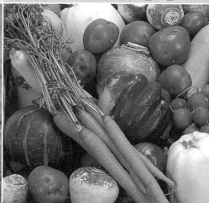

NUTRITION *for* HEALTH, STRENGTH, & LIFELONG VITALITY

I n my previous books, *Pushing Yourself to Power, The Miracle Seven,* and the *60 Day Personal Power Health and Fitness Journal,* I outlined complete nutritional strategies for the expressed purpose of losing excess body fat on the hurry-up while giving your body everything necessary to build lithe, beautifully sculpted muscle. In this book, however, I focus on helping you discover for yourself the best and most optimum way to feed and nourish yourself for health, strength, and vibrant lifelong vitality. So with this in mind, please read on.

Just about everyone knows and scientific research supports the fact that what we eat affects every aspect of our lives. Think about it. That means that what we ingest affects our physical energy, our mind and moods, and our longevity. Thus, it's obvious that we need to pay attention to what, when, and how we eat.

Yet I want to warn you about making diet and nutrition too great a preoccupation. As my grandfather and Uncle Wally used to tell me, "If you become too obsessed and fanatical with purity and dietary discipline, you'll drive yourself nuts, Jackson. And the stress alone is gonna kill you."

So, friends, don't get lost in the details of good nutrition—how many calories this or that food has or whether the protein and carbohydrates are in perfectly balanced ratios. Instead, I recommend focusing on the *seven key nutritional principles* that follow in this chapter. But first, let's overview how your chosen nutritional strategy can impact both the length and quality of your life.

NUTRITION AND LONGEVITY

Some gerontologists suggest that longevity depends upon genetics. Others disagree. Studies of the diets, physical activities, and lifestyles of other cultures whose people live extremely long lives suggest that our genetic inheritance may create *a tendency* to live a longer or shorter life, but that we also have the ability to maximize our genetic potential through the choices we make.

My conclusions are based on the scientific research conducted by Dr. Kenneth Pelletier and Paul Bragg. Dr. Pelletier studied the Vilca-bamba people of Ecudorian Andes, the Hunza people of northern Pakistan, the Mabaan people of Sudan, the Abkhazian people in the former Soviet Union, and the Tarahumara Indians of northern Mexico (known for their foot races that last up to 100 miles and more). Each of these distinct groups is known for their longevity, with many men and women living well past the century mark. They are also well known for the complete lack of the degenerative diseases that are normally associated with "aging" in the industrialized Western countries of the world. In fact, some of these people are known to live well into the 115- to 120-year range without disabilities. So Dr. Pelletier deemed them worthy of serious study.

Perhaps most important of all was that Dr. Pelletier found that the same exact factors that contribute toward the *quantity* and energy of life also contribute to its *quality*. This is great news! After all, who wants to sign up for a long, slow, and painful decline, just creaking along for the last 50 or more years until you die? Certainly not me. On the other hand, when life is filled with joy and vitality, each day brings yet another opportunity to experience LIFE and all of its blessings to the fullest, which holds great appeal to me. Bottom line: Dr. Pelletier's research proved beyond all doubt that the most effective way to increase both the *quality* and *quantity* of life is through the nutritional choices we make.

SEVEN GOLDEN KEYS TO NUTRITIONAL FITNESS

The following guidelines do not require sudden changes in your lifestyle that cannot be maintained. To the contrary, abrupt changes have a way of changing back to bad old habits rather quickly. If you think I'm wrong about that, ask yourself how many New Year's resolutions you were ever able to maintain long term. Point made.

Instead, these practices involve a gradual adaptation to a new and enlivening lifestyle as you pay attention to what you eat and how you feel afterward. The goal is to find the foods that work best for you and to avoid the extremes of self-denial and self-indulgence. You create this lifestyle by applying the following principles.

1. EAT BETTER FOOD WHILE CONSUMING FEWER CALORIES

Moderate, systematic under eating with higher quality food may be the single most important dietary practice of all. Long-lived peoples consume 1,800 to 2,000 calories per day by contrast to the average Westerner's 3,200 to 3,500 calories per day. Even more important is the source of the calories. For instance, just one piece of pecan pie contains 800 calories, and almost all those calories come from refined sugar and fat. Contrast that to a large Granny Smith apple that has only 100 calories and far greater nutritional value, and it is easy to see the difference. Nonetheless, please note that this practice of systematic under eating does *not* apply to growing children, people with very lean body types, pregnant or lactating women, those with high metabolic rates or caloric expenditures, such as athletes or laborers, and certainly not for those with eating disorders.

2. DON'T OVER CONSUME PROTEIN

Here in the U.S., many people worry about getting enough protein. However, the reality is that many people are consuming protein far in excess of their body's needs. High protein intake places tremendous stress on the internal organs to process it as well as makes a person feel lethargic and sluggish. This is due in part to the fact that protein and fat literally go hand in hand when it comes to consuming large amounts of animal protein.

One of the things Dr. Pelletier discovered was that virtually all of the long-lived peoples consume about half the protein of the average Westerner, with the vast majority of them being near vegetarians whose protein comes mainly from grains, legumes, and dairy products. These people almost never eat red meat and only small amounts of fish or poultry, yet the benefits are undeniable. Long-lived people have far lower cholesterol levels, almost no coronary disease, and virtually no osteoporosis. So they're obviously on to something that can make a huge difference in how we look and feel.

3. ENJOY A WIDE VARIETY OF NOURISHING FOODS

Whenever possible buy organically grown natural foods and stay away from those that are genetically altered. For instance, many of today's large farming conglomerates use genetically altered grains in order to maximize grain yields. As a result, each kernel of wheat is perfectly uniform and has the exact same amino acid profile. But if you were to visit one of the organic wheat farms in the Caucasus Mountains in Russia, home of the long-lived Hunza people, you'd find something totally different. Here the wheat fields contain different sizes and colors of plants, genetically diverse wheat with a variety of amino acids that combine into complete protein. This is also true of organically grown wheat here in the U.S. and Canada. This principle applies to far more than wheat, of course. Anyone who eats a varied diet of different organically grown seasonal fruits, vegetables, grains, and legumes is guaranteed abundant protein, vitamins, and minerals.

4. TRUST YOUR INSTINCTS AND DON'T BE AFRAID TO EXPERIMENT

It has been documented in many research experiments conducted by nutritional scientists that young children, when exposed to a variety of food groups over time, choose a well-balanced diet with the nutrients they need. Unfortunately, few of us were ever allowed to trust our instincts, relying instead on what we were taught by our parents, sold through advertising, or picked up in theories from a variety of diet books that often were contradictory. The truth is that our instincts have often been distorted through no fault of our own, whether that involved a limited selection of food in the home while growing up, television advertising, or peer pressure to conform.

But that was then and this is now, and as an adult, you can take control and do something about it. You can sharpen your instincts through exercise and fasting, as well as by adding and subtracting different kinds of foods from your dietary strategy and then paying close attention to how you feel after eating. This is one of the surest ways of combining natural instinct with awareness and discovering the optimal diet that is right for you. Bottom line: you don't need anyone's permission. You can trust your body over any harebrained theories or systems.

5. PRACTICE PERIODIC CLEANSING OR FASTING

One of the greatest physical culturists who ever lived was Paul Bragg, N.D., who died prematurely as a result of a surfing accident at the age of 95. As noted in the history section, Dr. Bragg was a powerfully built man who practiced Isometric Contraction and taught it to his students worldwide in his numerous books and seminars. In addition to "cutting edge" exercise for lifelong health and youthfulness, Dr. Bragg was also a world-class nutritionist who believed in and taught the almost miraculous benefits of periodic fasting. In fact, fasting, or going without food for one or more days while drinking plenty of water and fruit juices, is a time-honored practice in nearly every spiritual tradition. For example, the prophets Moses and Elijah as well as the Lord Jesus Christ completed 40-day fasts according to Scripture.

Fasting provides a rest for the digestive system, generates a physical cleansing, detoxifying effect, improves immune function, affords extra time for prayer, reflection, and contemplation, and relieves the subconscious mind of *fear* by providing the secure knowledge that if you ever have to go without food for days, you can do so. Nonetheless, in spite of its myriad health benefits, fasting is not recommended for growing children, pregnant and lactating disorders, or lean ectomorphic body types with high metabolisms. Nor is it a weight-loss method.

Before starting a fast, be sure to read Dr. Paul Bragg's *The Miracle of Fasting* or *Fasting Made Simple* by Paula White. If you have any doubts or medical problems, consult a health professional familiar with fasting.

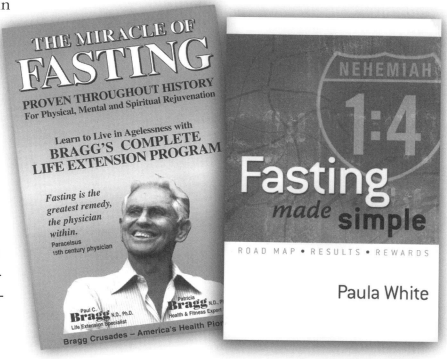

6. ENJOY MORE RAW FRUITS AND VEGETABLES

Increasing the proportion of fresh, uncooked vegetables and fruits in your diet provides unprocessed nutrients in their most direct form, with a complete array of live enzymes that help you assimilate the food you eat. These high-moisture content foods also provide fiber necessary for good elimination. Eating mostly or exclusively raw foods naturally promotes weight loss, while insuring high-quality nutrition and vitality. Eating raw fruits and vegetables exclusively for a period of time has much the same cleansing effect as periodic fasting.

7. PAY ATTENTION TO HOW YOU EAT AND DRINK

How you eat is nearly as important as what you eat. This was a point driven home in the world famous Charles Atlas Dynamic Tension Body Building Course, and it is just as true today. Mr. Atlas was quick to point out that a few simple habits can enhance your digestion and help you derive the most value from the food you consume. One of his key principles was to chew your food very well and to breathe very deeply while eating, savoring the taste, texture, and aroma as you chew. He literally advised to chew each bite as though it was the only one you'd have all day. Put down your knife and fork between each bite and allow your body to relax and enjoy. (Don't worry, I haven't succeeded at this one either.)

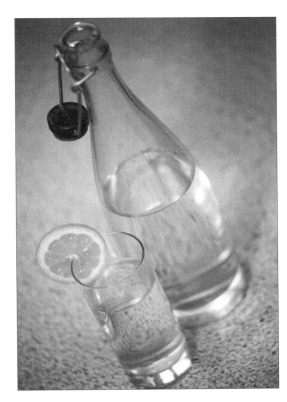

Ultimately, just as with your practice of Isometric exercise, you are the final authority over how you feed your body, and you have to find what works best for you. Always favor experimentation over rigid rules prescribed by someone else. Remember, just as with your Isometric exercises, good nutrition involves lifelong learning and application, and no other person could possibly know what is best for you, so it's important that you become your own most reliable expert.

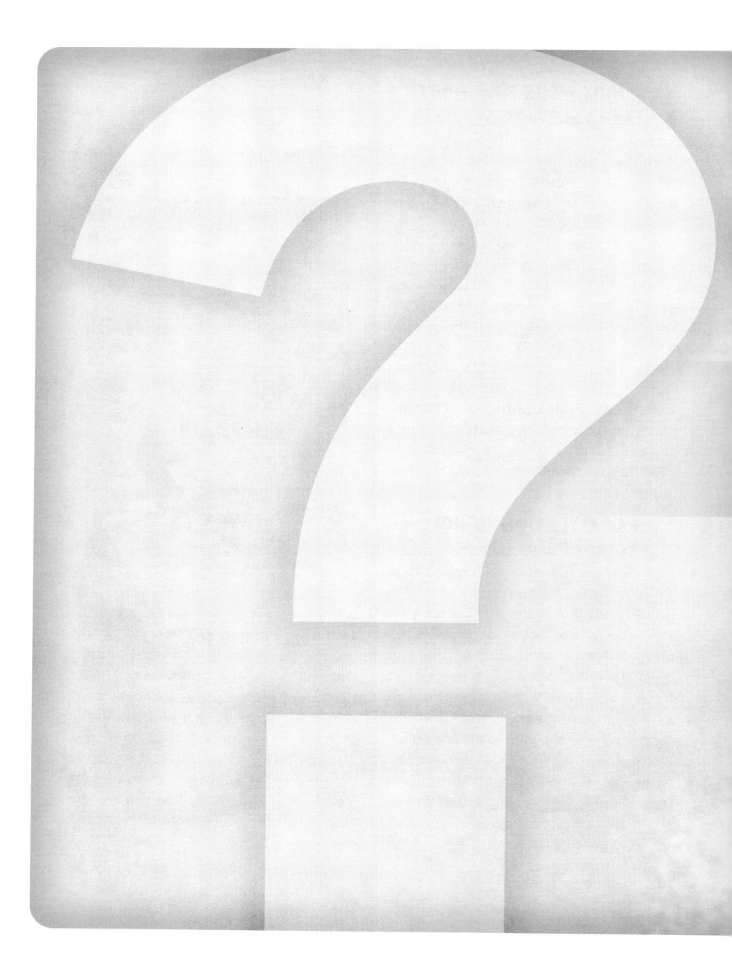

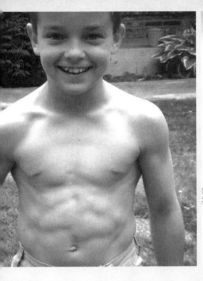
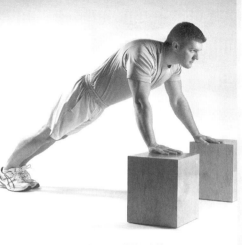
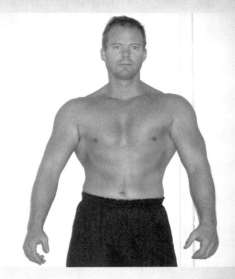

ISOMETRIC Q & A's

*Answers for the Questions You Have
Now or May Have in the Future*

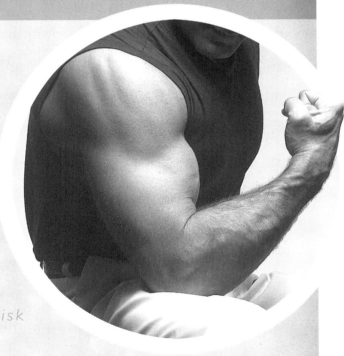

*How many variations of Isometric
exercises are there?*

*Will Isometric Contraction give me
a bodybuilder's physique?*

*Do Isometrics pose the same risk
of injury as other forms
of strength training?*

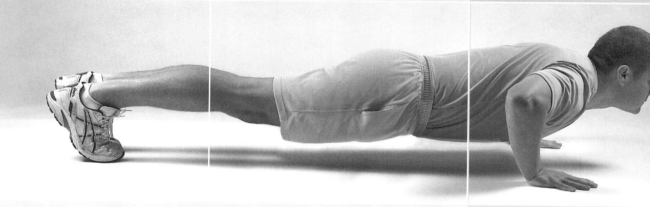

CHAPTER FOUR

ISOMETRIC Q&A'S

Answers for the Questions You Have Now or May Have in the Future

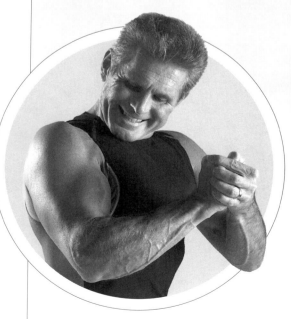

In the next several pages you'll find more than a dozen of the most frequently asked questions that I have received regarding Isometric Contraction. Because they have been asked by so many over the past three years, it's obvious to me that these are in fact the most important ones to answer.

How long should each Isometric Contraction be held for maximum effectiveness?

The length of an Isometric Contraction is totally dependent upon the level of intensity. The greater the intensity—in other words, the closer you are to exerting 100 percent of your available strength—the shorter the duration.

According to Dr. Theodore Hettinger, who performed the original Isometric Studies during the late '40s and '50s with Dr. E. A. Müeller at the Max Planck Institute in Dortmund, Germany, if you are using 100 percent of your strength, the contraction needs to be held for only 1 to 2 seconds. If your muscles are contracting at 40 to 50 percent of maximum perceived strength, a duration of 15 to 20 seconds was recommended by Hettinger.

In recent years, Strongman Steve Justa has coined the term *Aerobic Isometrics* and recommends contractions of 35 percent of perceived strength to be held from 2 to 5 minutes. I have several friends who have tried this method with excellent results.

The duration or time of contraction is strictly dependent upon the intensity of the contraction.

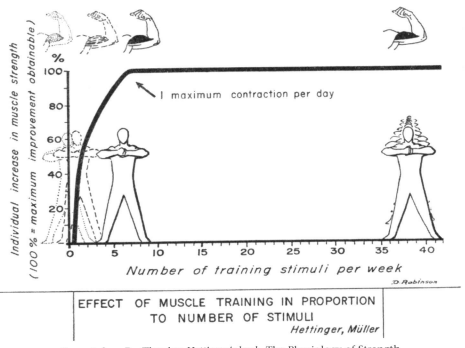

Figure 5 from Dr. Theodore Hettinger's book, The Physiology of Strength

Will Isometric Contraction give me a bodybuilder's physique?

. . . .

While Isometric Contraction can be invaluable in building superior strength and helping you achieve a beautifully sculpted musculature, there are other factors besides exercise alone that determine to what extent you develop your physique. But to answer your question directly, no, Isometric Contraction alone will not make you look like a bodybuilder juiced up on steroids. It flat out won't happen.

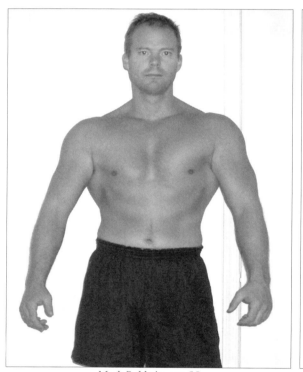

Mark Baldwin, age 38

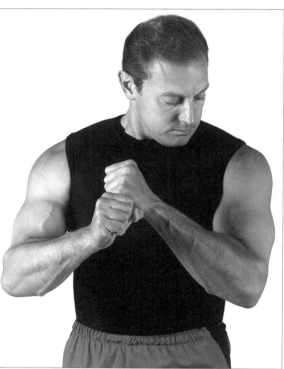

Chris Rezny, age 42

On the other hand, by spending 30 to 45 minutes each day, combining 10 to 15 minutes of Isometrics with our Power Calisthenics and DVR/DSR exercises, you can achieve a beautifully sculpted, perfectly balanced physique as is exemplified by my friends and students, personal trainer Mark Baldwin and Chris Rezny (pictured above). As you can see, both men are very muscular—not in the rococo, overly developed, almost freakish manner of contemporary bodybuilders who are, in fact, juiced up on steroids, but in the practical way an athletic animal such as a thoroughbred racehorse is muscular. In other words, you're going to look like a beautifully conditioned athlete.

Is it true that Isometrics can cause a dangerous elevation in blood pressure?

Over the past two years, I have received numerous e-mails asking me this question. For this reason, I have written a chapter that deals with this issue that begins on page 104. Nevertheless, here's a brief answer for the sake of brevity.

All forms of strenuous exertion will cause a short-term elevation in blood pressure. Even raking leaves, shoveling snow, or changing a tire will do it. The real issues surrounding the blood pressure question are (A.) Do Isometrics cause a sudden and dangerous elevation in blood pressure? and (B.) Do Isometrics cause a long-term and permanent elevation in blood pressure even when one is not engaged in strenuous activities?

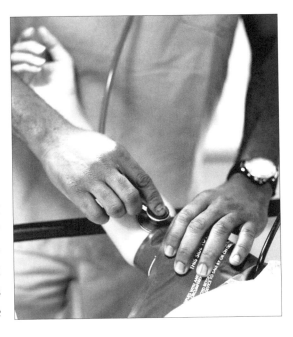

The answer to (A.) is that if you were to perform sudden and extremely intense Isometric Contractions without slowly building the tension in your muscles until you achieve peak contraction (in other words, you suddenly *jolt* yourself into an ultra-high intensity contraction), the answer is *yes!* You could cause a sudden and unsafe elevation in blood pressure, not to mention the very real probability of tearing muscles at the attachment point to their tendons. Such an action is one that I consider to be suicidally stupid. However, if you follow the Isometric Contraction protocols that I have outlined in this book, the answer is a resounding *no!*

The answer to (B.) is also *no!* In fact, if you go to page 108, I provide information about Isometric Contraction being used clinically to *lower* blood pressure.

BOTTOM LINE: responsible implementation of Isometric Contraction will only benefit you.

How often do I need to train with Isometrics in order to achieve maximum results?

This is a great question that I'm frequently asked, and one that the researchers at the Max Planck Institute tested and retested hundreds of time. The results of their research were first published in English in 1961 with the release of Dr. Theodore Hettinger's *Physiology of Strength*. The following quote is the answer he gave to the question of "how often," but before you read it, let me clue you in on the meaning of the word *abscissa* (I didn't have a clue as to what it means). *Abscissa* means "the horizontal coordinate of a point in a plane Cartesian coordinate system obtained by measuring parallel to the x-axis."

"In Figure 5 the results of many experiments on many subjects are combined. The number of training stimuli is shown in the abscissa; the increase in muscle strength in percentage of the maximum improvement obtainable is given in the ordinate. It was found that the maximum increase in muscle strength was obtained with one training stimulus per day. Administering this same stimulus up to seven times a day

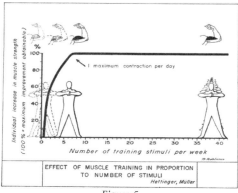

Figure 5

did not increase muscle strength any more rapidly. Also several maximum contractions one after the other (as many as twelve contractions in a one-second rhythm) did not increase the strength any faster than only one contraction. It therefore seems that the muscle, after one training stimulus during any one day, is unresponsive to any further training stimulus on the same day. When training sessions were held only each second day, the increase in strength was about 80 percent; with two training sessions per week, the increase was about 60 percent, and when training sessions were held only once a week, only about 40 percent of the improvement in strength was obtained as compared with the once-a-day regime; and one training stimulus every 14 days produced no change at all in muscle strength."

As you can see from the results of the researchers at the Max Planck Institute, the best all-around results were achieved with *one* daily Isometric Contraction. Performing more repetitions, while not detrimental, offered no additional benefit for the acquisition of strength. This was also true of Isometric Pulse Training, where as many as twelve one-second maximum contractions were repeated in a one-second pulse rhythm. Bottom line: for the acquisition of *strength only,* a frequency of one contraction daily gave the best results.

Can I achieve a complete workout with Isometrics alone?

For strength building and muscle sculpting, *yes!* But for all-around athletic fitness, *no!* Let me explain.

There are seven components to lifelong athletic strength and fitness. They are strength, flexibility, endurance (muscular and cardiovascular), balance, coordination, reaction time (speed), and aesthetics (how your body looks).

Isometric Contraction will develop strength and aesthetics particularly well, and it will *certainly make you strong* so that your body can easily handle other exercises that improve cardio/muscular endurance, flexibility, balance, coordination, and speed. In fact, Strongman Steve Justa, for whom I have the utmost of respect, is adamant that Isometrics are superior for the procurement of speed. Even so, as with any other form of exercise, from my perspective, Isometric Contraction is best used in combination with other types of exercise for a complete workout.

Nonetheless, I don't hesitate to recommend Isometric Contraction as a stand-alone system of exercise if someone simply has no time for anything else. As I view it, one has everything to gain and nothing to lose by implementing Isometrics into their lives. After all, the vast majority of these exercises can be integrated into your daily schedule at random moments throughout the day without it even being noticed by other people.

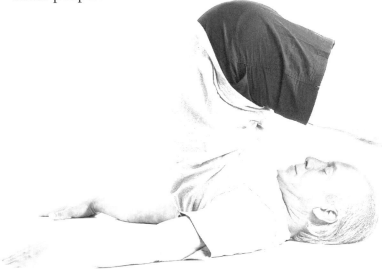

Do Isometrics pose the same risk of injury as other forms of strength training?

If followed exactly as instructed in this book, *absolutely not!* In fact, Isometric Contraction as outlined in this book is far and away the safest form of strength building that one can follow. But here's the deal. You need to follow the method *exactly* as outlined in this book. As I mentioned previously, if you were to suddenly *jolt* yourself into an intense contraction with no gradual buildup of tension, you'd be asking for trouble. And if that were the case, it would not be Isometric Contraction that is to blame but stupidity.

One other proof of the safety of sensibly applied Isometric Contraction is the fact that when Drs. Hettinger and Müeller began conducting their experiments in 1946 at the Max Plank Institute, it was for the purpose of discovering the best, safest, and most adaptable methods of strength training to be used in helping injured soldiers to rehabilitate injuries sustained in WWII and return to normal life.

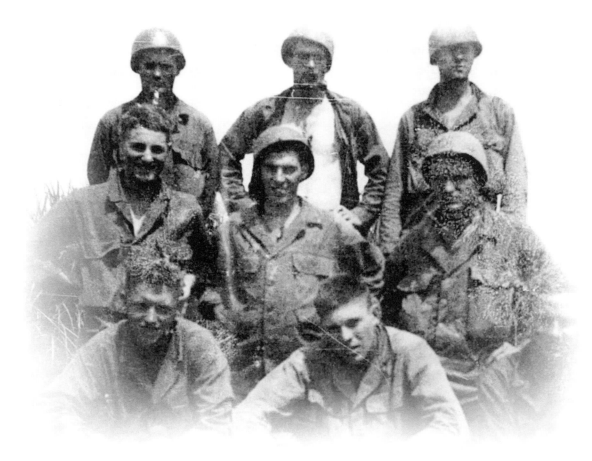

Did Charles Atlas teach a course in Isometrics?

I've already answered this question in Chapter 2, but here goes.

Ever since I was a kid, I can't begin to count the number of articles that I have read where a self-professed authority on strength and fitness has stated that Charles Atlas taught a system of Isometric exercises. Whenever I read that assertion, it automatically tells me two things. One, the expert doesn't know what he's talking about. And, two, he has never read the *Atlas Dynamic Tension Course*. Atlas's course taught self-resistance exercises that utilized one set of muscles working in opposition against another through various ranges of motion as well as carefully selected power calisthenics. He did not teach Isometric (static or motionless) Contraction as it was known or taught during the late 1950s and throughout the '60s.

In fact, I have several copies of the *Atlas Dynamic Tension Course* dating from the '30s, '40s, '50s, '60s, and '70s, with one dating back to its inception in 1922, and the exercises never changed. Don't misunderstand my point. I'm not saying the Atlas exercises could not be utilized in an Isometric fashion. In fact, I already told you about my uncle Milo doing Atlas exercises in that fashion. My point is that Mr. Atlas never taught them that way.

So the next time you read a so-called expert who says that Charles Atlas taught a system of Isometric exercises, you may as well disregard whatever else he is saying, because he hasn't done his homework. And if he's wrong about that, how can you be sure he is correct about anything else?

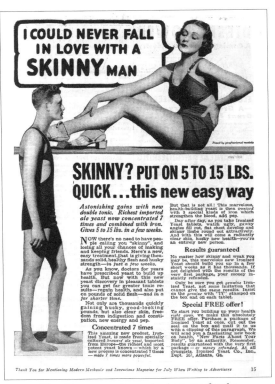

The skinny guy always had an eye for the beautiful girls in the 1930s' advertising.

How many variations of Isometric exercises are there?

In recent years, several authors and physiologists have begun to refer to virtually all forms of motionless exercise as "Isometrics"—for instance, "core" stabilization exercises, such as Planks, yoga, Pilates, and Callanetics. These and other similar exercise systems are ones that place an emphasis on holding specific body postures and alignment in motionless positions against the force of gravity alone for up to several minutes at a time.

Because so many "experts" are trying to lump all these motionless exercises into the category of "Isometrics," I want to clarify and define the three types of "Isometric" exercise that we will be using in this book. They are:

I. *CIC* or Classic Isometric Contraction

II. *SIP* or Static Isometric Postures

III. *PCIP* or Peak Contraction Isometric Power Flex

I. CLASSIC ISOMETRIC CONTRACTION

In the history section of this book, I referred to the Isometric Contraction experiments that were conducted at Springfield College in Massachusetts during the 1920s as well as those conducted by Dr. E. A. Müeller and Dr. Theodore Hettinger at the Max Planck Institute in Dortmund, Germany, utilizing more than 5,000 volunteers from 1946 to 1960. It was from Hettinger and Müeller's ground-breaking discoveries that Isometric Contraction was verified and quantified for the first time, using human test subjects. As stated previously, the results were nothing less than astounding.

For the sake of brevity, throughout this text we will refer to Classic Isometric Contraction as the *willful* contraction of a specific muscle or muscle group against an immovable force, object, or another muscle group at ultra-high intensity. In other words, *Classic Isometric Contraction* is the term that will be used when we refer to contracting our muscles against or in opposition to something else with such intensity that no movement is possible. For all intents and purposes, the muscles are in a deadlock.

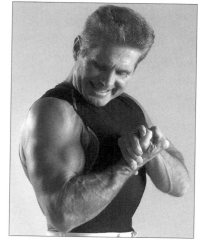

II. STATIC ISOMETRIC POSTURES

In yoga and the martial arts, as well as in certain physical therapy exercises, there is a type of Isometric exercise that utilizes the muscles as stabilizers against the effects of gravity. The Bridge and Planks are two primary examples. In these instances, the muscles are not contracting against any other force or an immovable object, but they are used isometrically to maintain proper body alignment.

This is also true for certain combination Isometric/Isotonic (or dynamic) exercises—for instance, when you perform push-ups in perfect form as you see Gregory performing in the photos below and on the two pages that follow. It is Isometric stabilization of the "core" muscles that allows him to maintain a straight back from his shoulders to his heels. So group II, Static Isometric Postures is the term used when we are performing Isometric stabilization exercises or Isotonic exercises requiring Isometric stabilization.

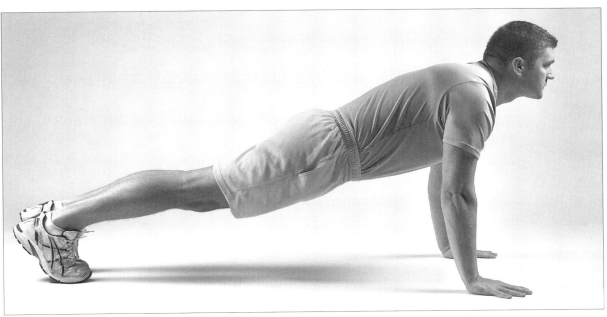

STANDARD PUSH-UPS

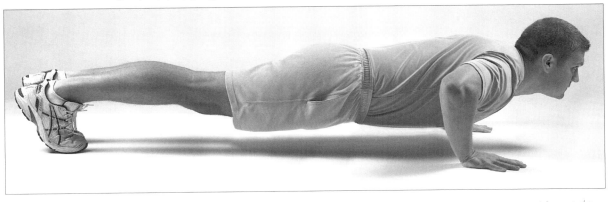

continued»

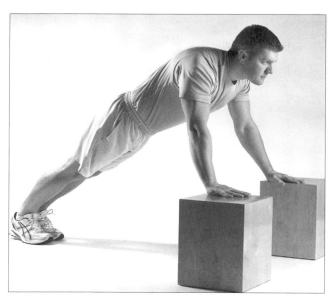
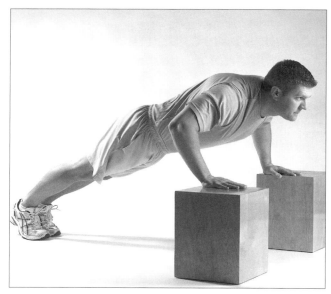

ATLAS PUSH-UPS

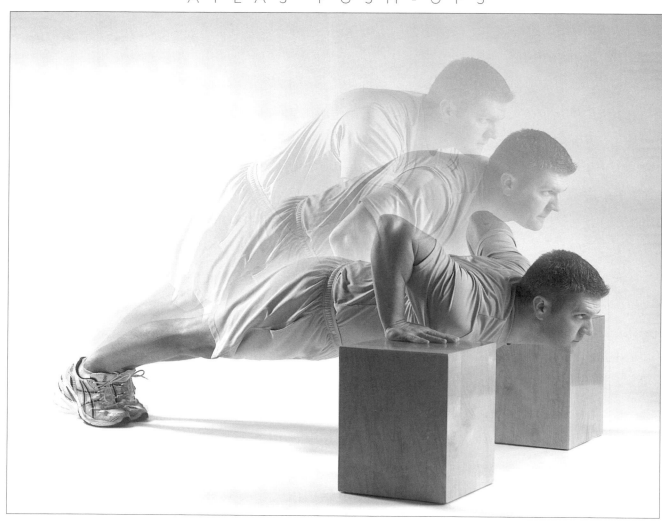

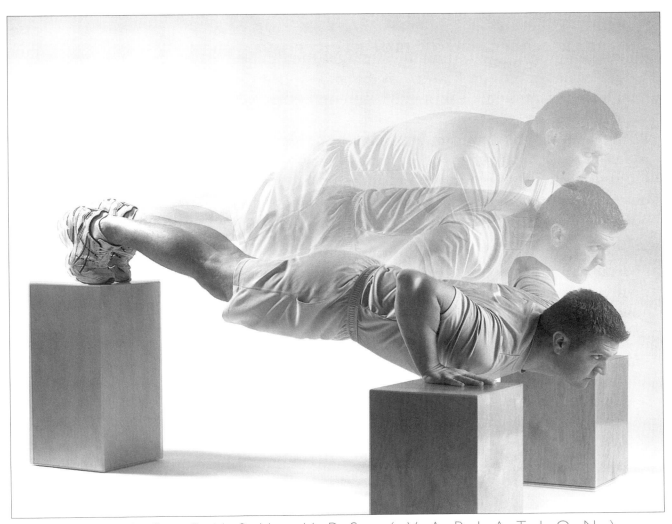

ATLAS PUSH-UPS (VARIATION)

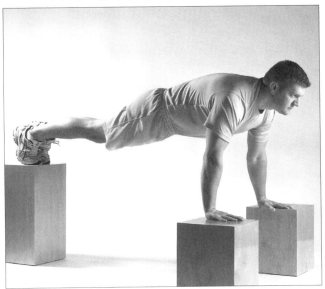

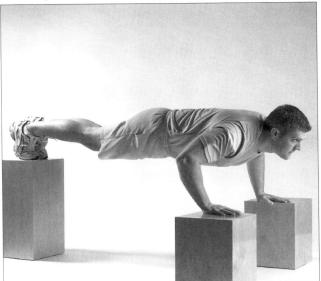

III. PEAK CONTRACTION ISOMETRIC POWER FLEX

Peak Contraction Isometric Power Flex is the term we use to refer to exercises where we intentionally contract our muscles with as much intensity as we can possibly engage, such as in the biceps pose you see pictured. As you will see, these Peak Contraction Isometric Power Flex contractions allow for incredible muscle sculpting and contouring, as well as the ability to control every muscle group at will. It is somewhat similar to Classic Isometric Contraction but does not employ contracting our muscles against an outside force or an immovable object. The intensity of these contractions depends solely on one's own ability to contract with *maximum intensity.*

An example of a Peak Contraction Isometric Power Flex is what professional bodybuilders use in their posing routines. These men and women literally exhaust themselves in just a few short minutes with their posing routines because of the intensity they put into their flexing movements. So much so that emergency medical staff are on hand to administer oxygen in case of a coronary—*and, no, I'm not joking.*

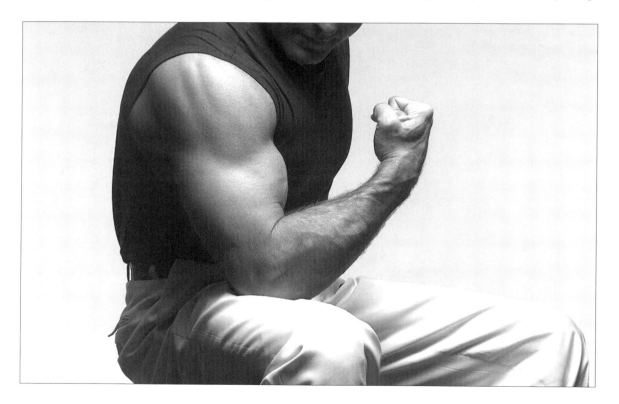

Will Isometrics make it possible for me to lift heavy weights?

I've been asked this question many times, and the answer is far more complicated than a simple yes or no. As stated consistently throughout this book, Isometric Contraction, when properly applied, can and will dramatically enhance muscular strength. However, lifting heavy weights is a skill that requires not only strength but balance, coordination, speed, and timing.

Just as you cannot realistically expect Isometric Contraction alone to help you hit more home runs unless you hone your batting skills in a batting cage to develop the rudiments of a flawless swing, including enhanced speed, timing, and hand/eye coordination, so you need to develop the elements of balance, coordination, speed, and timing to excel at weightlifting.

For instance, Alexander Zass, the Russian strongman whom I referred to in the history section, was exceptionally strong as a result of his Isometric Contraction exercise system. He was so strong, in fact, that the mightiest weightlifters of his time could not match him at either bar bending or chain breaking. Yet, Zass, of his own admission, was not talented as a weightlifter and did not perform well at it.

BOTTOM LINE: Isometric Contraction can and will help you to become phenomenally strong, but by itself it will not enhance other athletic attributes. You need to develop the other requisite skills to become a superior athlete, whether you're talking about hitting baseballs, playing golf, or lifting heavy weights. Hence, the need to incorporate other forms of exercise for increased athletic conditioning.

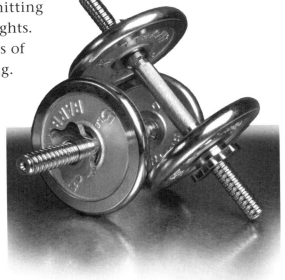

Here's my question to someone who wants to lift heavy weights: why do you want to expose yourself to a source of exercise that has resulted in tens of thousands suffering from bad elbows, bad wrists, severe lower back and knee pain, as well as destroyed joints, ligaments, and tendons? It doesn't make any sense when Isometric Contraction delivers superb results while protecting the whole body.

In simple English, what is the concept behind Isometric Contraction? And why is it so effective?

To get to the last repetition—**FIRST**! Let me explain what I mean by that. Let's just say that someone performs an exercise for one set of 12 repetitions to reach the point of fatigue, where he or she simply cannot perform one more repetition. Now, from the perspective of strength building only, ask yourself why the first 11 repetitions were necessary. Answer: to fatigue the muscles for that final hardest and most effective repetition. In other words, the first 11 repetitions were used to exhaust the muscle for the performance of the last most challenging repetition.

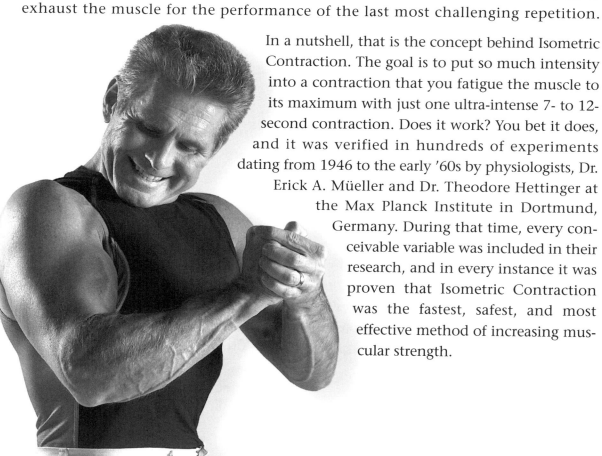

In a nutshell, that is the concept behind Isometric Contraction. The goal is to put so much intensity into a contraction that you fatigue the muscle to its maximum with just one ultra-intense 7- to 12-second contraction. Does it work? You bet it does, and it was verified in hundreds of experiments dating from 1946 to the early '60s by physiologists, Dr. Erick A. Müeller and Dr. Theodore Hettinger at the Max Planck Institute in Dortmund, Germany. During that time, every conceivable variable was included in their research, and in every instance it was proven that Isometric Contraction was the fastest, safest, and most effective method of increasing muscular strength.

John, my son, Adam, is 10 years old. Do you think it is safe for him to follow the Isometric training methods that you have outlined in Pushing Yourself to Power?
—Jerry S.

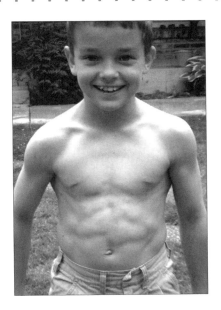

That's a good question, Jerry, and one that I have been frequently asked. As you know from reading *Pushing Yourself to Power,* I literally started training with these methods when I was 10 years old, after I got the stuffing knocked out of me by a gigantic 13-year-old bully. (He's probably still singing soprano today some 44 years later after my brother was finished with him.) The truth is, these methods are perfect for young boys/men to learn and master, particularly as they are going through puberty. Take for example these three photos of my 11-year-old nephew R.J. As you can clearly see in these photos of R.J. performing his uncle's exercises, they have only helped him and enhanced his athletic ability. And if I say so myself, R.J. has a great physique and great self-confidence as well as muscle mastery for an 11-year-old.

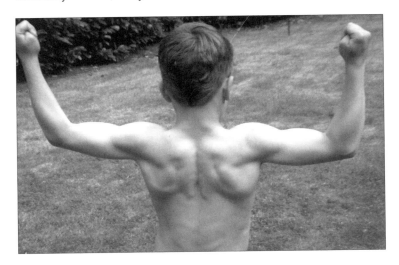

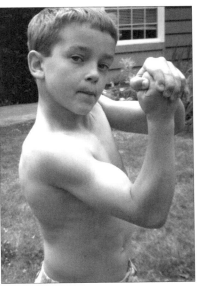

Not as we teach it. Static Contraction Training (SCT) is a method whereby one holds enormous amounts of weight in positions of greatest strength. No attempt is made to lift the weight or move it through a full range of motion. When I say that the weight is held or supported in specific positions of greatest strength for 15 to 30 seconds, I am giving you the entire method in a nutshell.

This method was made popular by Pete Sisco and John R. Little and endorsed by motivational guru Anthony Robbins, who has had Sisco and Little appear with him on various programs (neither man is built like an adonis). The claims for the method are outlandish and not based upon fact. I have known four men who have used this method exclusively, and in each case the results were disappointing.

For instance, I have a friend in Canada by the name of Dave Walmsley, who is a fire-fighter by trade. He is also an expert in self-defense and teaches an excellent self-defense system called Canadian Combato. Dave told me about an 8-month experiment he conducted utilizing the SCT method exactly as outlined by Sisco and Little. For instance, when he began his experiment with the exercises suggested, he started at around 200 pounds for the seated shoulder press and eventually was able to use more than 350 pounds for a timed static hold. On the bench press, he began at around 350 pounds (at close-to-complete extension, the position of greatest strength) and worked up to more than 450 pounds for a timed static hold. He even got to the point where he was using 2,200 pounds on the leg press for the full time limit.

But…and this is where it all unraveled for him…prior to static contraction training, Dave was incredibly strong and fit in an athletically functional way. He could perform over 100 push-ups nonstop, 20 chin-ups nonstop, and had even performed 3 sets of 10 repetition chin-ups with 30 pounds tied to his waist. But at the end of 8 months of SCT, he struggled to complete 40 push-ups and found 10 body weight chin-ups to be difficult. In addition, he said that his strength through the full range of motion on certain standard weight training exercises had not improved, and in some cases had even decreased from what it was prior to his SCT experiment. Bottom line: although he did add considerable strength to hold or support weight, it did not in any way improve his athletic functional strength or physique.

In addition to Dave, I have known three other men who also followed the same SCT protocols. Their experiences were virtually identical in that they all added tremendously to the weight they could hold in one position. But they *all* lost "enduring

continued»

strength" and were very disappointed with their overall results. This was particularly so because not one of them had improved the aesthetics of their physiques by using the SCT method.

Does that mean that SCT is worthless? Not if supporting weight is something you like to do. But in terms of strength and muscle building, it won't even compare to the results you can achieve performing Isometric Contractions as we teach them. Why? Because if range of motion, strength, and muscle sculpting are the goal, it is imperative that the muscles be contracted as powerfully as possible in the stretched (elongated), mid contraction, and fully contracted (peak) positions. Holding or supporting a weight where you are not actively engaged in trying to move it produces only one-dimensional strength. Then again, if that is what you enjoy, go to it.

question #13

John, I'm 6'1" and weigh 145 pounds. Will Isometrics help me gain solid muscular weight? I'd like to add about 40 pounds to my frame.

It all depends. If you have an extremely high metabolism or are naturally thin (ectomorphic), it may take some period of time before you reach your desired weight. As stated elsewhere in this book, Isometrics when combined with right Isotonics can dramatically enhance your physique—no doubt about it! But it still isn't a magic wand.

Weight gaining, particularly gaining muscular weight, takes time for many individuals. Now, there are some wonderful weight gaining formulas available at health food stores, and some are excellent. By that I mean they even taste great (unlike when I was in my teens and the only stuff available, such as Hoffman's Protein From the Sea, tasted as though it had been recycled through a horse).

The other thing you can do is to eat more frequently and drink large quantities of certified organic raw milk, if it is available to you. My uncles used that method right out of Charles Atlas's course in the 1930s, and they swore by it.

Other than that, well, I knew one guy who went on an every three hour eating-to-gain-weight schedule for football. He even set his alarm clock to wake him in the middle of the night in order to eat. Did it work? Yes, he got as big as a house, but it certainly wasn't all muscle. Was that a healthy thing to do? Only in your dreams.

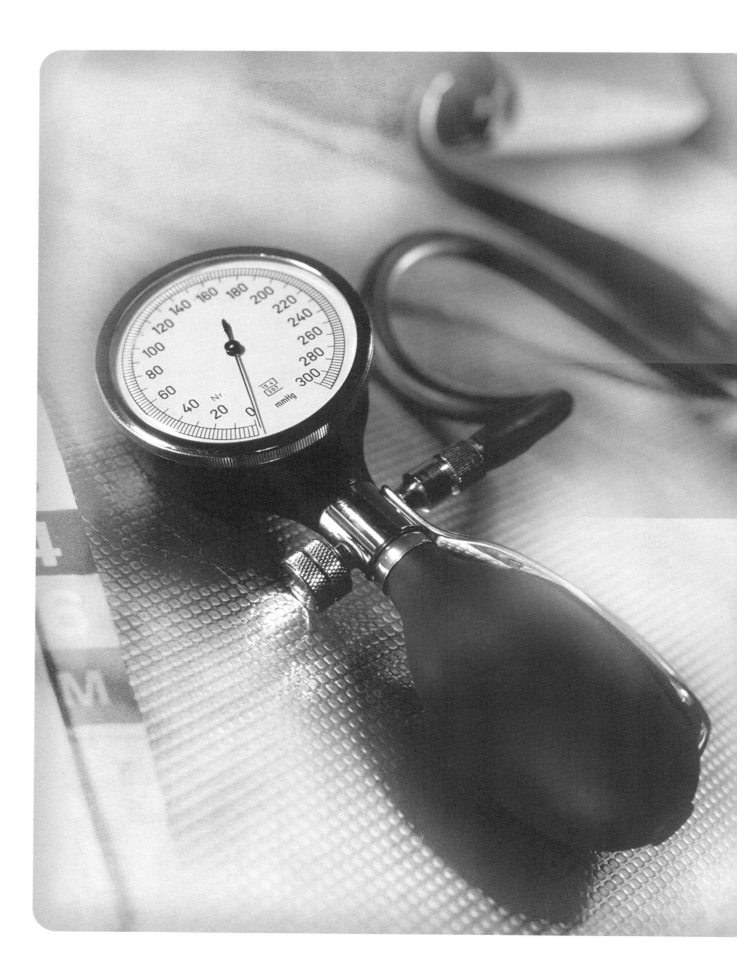

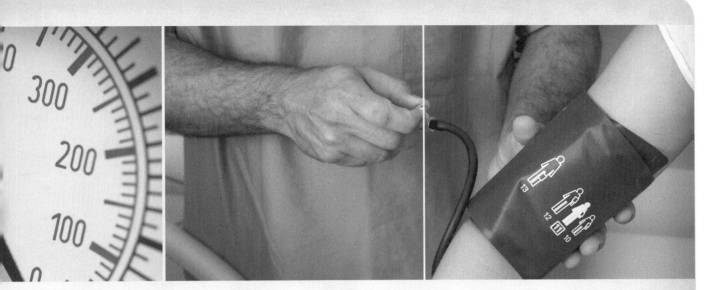

CHAPTER FIVE

BLOOD PRESSURE AND
ISOMETRIC CONTRACTION

*Lowering Blood Pressure Naturally,
Safely, and Permanently*

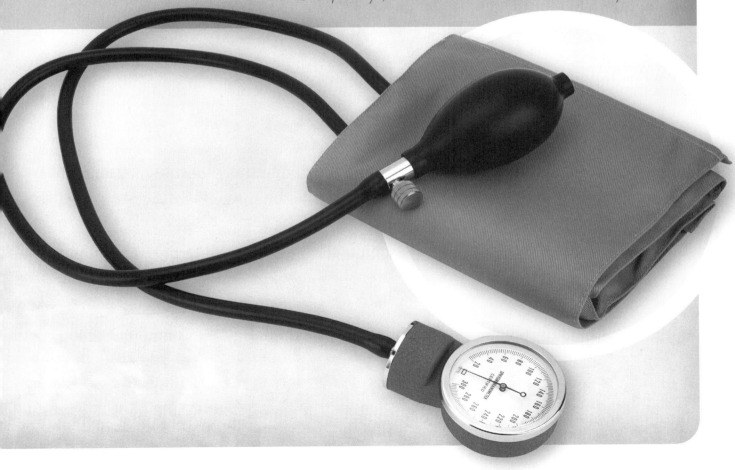

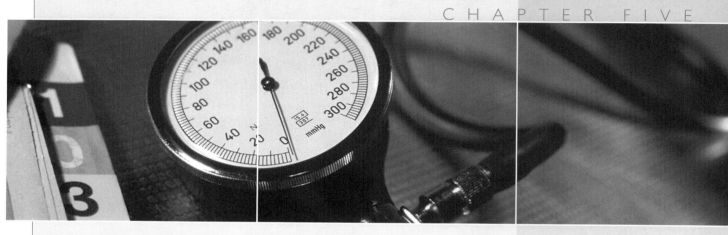

BLOOD PRESSURE AND ISOMETRIC CONTRACTION

Lowering Blood Pressure Naturally, Safely, and Permanently

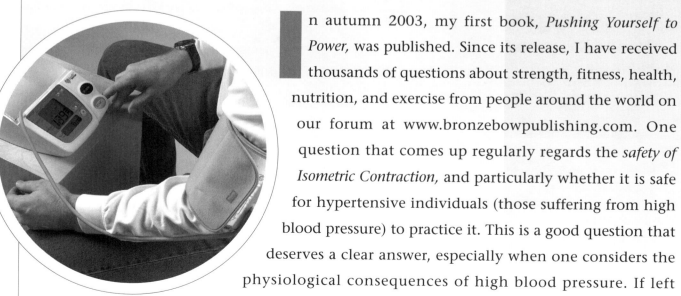

n autumn 2003, my first book, *Pushing Yourself to Power,* was published. Since its release, I have received thousands of questions about strength, fitness, health, nutrition, and exercise from people around the world on our forum at www.bronzebowpublishing.com. One question that comes up regularly regards the *safety of Isometric Contraction,* and particularly whether it is safe for hypertensive individuals (those suffering from high blood pressure) to practice it. This is a good question that deserves a clear answer, especially when one considers the physiological consequences of high blood pressure. If left untreated, hypertension carries a three-fold increase (300 percent) in the risk for developing coronary artery disease and a sevenfold increase (700 percent) for the likelihood of developing a stroke or aneurysm. Bottom line: high blood pressure is not to be taken lightly or fooled around with.

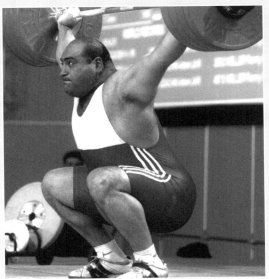

All forms of extreme exertion can elevate blood pressure to dangerous levels... especially if one is holding their breath.

WHAT HYPERTENSION IS

Defined as a chronically elevated blood pressure greater than 140/90 mm Hg, hypertension is diagnosed by taking noninvasive measurements of the resting blood pressure on two or more occasions. Normal resting blood pressure in apparently healthy individuals averages 120/80 mm Hg. The first number, 120, represents the pressure against the 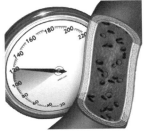 artery walls when the heart contracts and is called *systolic blood pressure*. The second number, 80, is the pressure against the artery walls during the resting phase (between heartbeats) and is called *diastolic blood pressure*. The difference between these two pressures, the <u>mean</u> <u>arterial</u> <u>pressure</u>, or MAP, represents the average blood pressure throughout the arterial system.

Specialized blood pressure sensors throughout the body regulate blood pressure and ensure that it does not fall too low, thus compromising adequate flow to tissues; or doesn't rise too high, thus increasing the work of the heart and over stressing the blood vessels. Generally, blood pressure is regulated in such a way that it rises and falls consistently with the demands of the body throughout the day. Occasionally, blood pressure control mechanisms throughout the body malfunction or are unable to compensate for the demands placed on the body, and one of the resulting conditions is hypertension.

HYPERTENSION AND ISOMETRIC EXERCISE

Now, let's get to the questions. First, does the practice of Isometric Contraction carry a substantial risk of elevating the blood pressure to unsafe levels during the actual time one is engaged in performing each contraction. And, second, does consistent practice of Isometric Contraction increase the risk of developing chronic hypertension even when one is not exercising? Here's the short answer to each one—*not if practiced the way we teach it in this book.* Let me explain what I mean by that statement. While it is true that all forms of strenuous exertion can and do raise blood pressure (sometimes to catastrophic levels), Isometric Contraction as we teach it with carefully controlled breathing does not pose the same risk or threat as does sudden and extreme exertion where the breath is held.

There are no new studies that deal specifically with Isometric Contraction and hypertension. However, there were two medical doctors, Rene Caillet, M.D., Clinical Professor at the University of Southern California School of Medicine, and Broino Kiveloff, M.D., Associate Chief of Rehabilitation Medicine at the New York Infirmary-Beekman Downtown Hospital, who used Isometric Contraction to treat hypertension with great success during the '60s, '70s, and '80s. In fact, Dr. Kiveloff was so sold on the benefits of full body Isometric Contraction (as he taught it) that he used it not only to treat hypertensives but also diabetics. In the 1986 *Journal of the Royal Society for the Promotion of Health,* Dr. Kiveloff was featured in an extensive article outlining exactly how his Isometric program for hypertensives could be used by diabetics with great benefit.

So what was Dr. Kiveloff's method? Hang tight because I am about to share it with you. His method was revealed in detail in an extensive article titled, "A 60-Second Shortcut to Vitality," that appeared in the February 1983 issue of *Prevention Magazine.* The article started with the question, "How does a person take action against age?" and was followed with the response, "There are many ways, but one takes less than a minute a day, costs nothing, and can be learned almost instantly. It's been shown to help fight high blood pressure, the major risk factor for heart attacks, stroke, and kidney disease, and now its inventor believes it can also retard age by the same mechanism."

"There are thousands of theories of aging," said Dr. Kiveloff. "This is a new one—the best one!" The article then went on to describe how strong, youthful, and young Dr. Kiveloff appeared to be even though he had been practicing medicine for 55 years, having begun in 1928! In addition to Dr. Kiveloff, the article also included references to his associate, Olive Huber, Ph.D., Professor Emeritus in the Department of Physiology at Hunter College, who had worked with Dr. Kiveloff since 1960 and was the co-developer of the technique.

The article featured references and quotes from numerous individuals who had achieved great benefits with the program and referenced clinical studies that had been conducted by Kiveloff and Huber respectively, all of which achieved and verified the same results—a dramatic decrease in resting blood pressure. So much so that many people no longer required blood pressure medication. One other side benefit was the dramatic improvement in posture, muscle tone, and general appearance that every man and woman who utilized the technique verified.

In fact, the article referred to one man who had been restricted to a salt-free diet when his doctor discovered that his blood pressure was 160/95. Every 3 months for 7 years this man had gone to his doctor for blood tests and checkups on his progress. Then, in just 5 to 8 weeks of following Dr. Kiveloff's Isometrics, his blood pressure fell to 120/80 and remained there. He was quoted in the article as saying, "It's so much more wonderful than taking medication. You have to go to the doctor only when you want to!"

Another individual story was that of a 65-year-old executive who stated he had not missed a single day of Isometrics since he began the program 7 years previously. When he began, his blood pressure was 185/105. In just a few months of Isometrics, it dropped to 130/70 and remained there. "I'm in awfully good shape, fit and flexible, and this is the only regular exercise I get," he told *Prevention Magazine*.

So what exactly was this extraordinary program? It's very simple, though it's important that it be done correctly. *The most important thing,* according to Dr. Kiveloff, *is to breathe normally doing Isometrics.* Also, observe the time limit: 6 to 7 seconds for each exercise. In medical jargon, the program's full name is "brief, maximal extensive Isometric exercise," Dr. Kiveloff stated, with an emphasis on *brief.* By counting out loud to easily keep track of your time, you can also maintain normal breathing.

HERE'S HOW IT'S DONE:

1. Stand in a relaxed position, arms hanging loose. *Don't* clench your fists or bend your elbows or joints.

2. Simultaneously tense all your muscles as tightly as possible, while breathing normally and counting out loud to seven. You might try tensing each muscle group separately—legs, arms, chest, abdomen, face, and then try tensing them all at once. When you do, you feel an immediate surge of warmth all over your body.

3. Relax and rest for a few seconds.

4. Repeat twice more for a total of 3 reps.

5. Do this 3 times a day (try morning, noon, and night).

That's all there is to Dr. Kiveloff's method for controlling hypertension by utilizing Isometric Contraction exercise. He stated he performed the exercise 4 or 5 times daily (a total of 12 to 15 repetitions) for added benefit. And, he added, though the original study was done with people exercising in a standing position, the exercise could also be done sitting or lying down. In fact, lying down before getting out of bed in the morning while practicing deep breathing was exactly how Dr. Rene Caillet, whom I referred to at the beginning of the chapter, taught the same exercise in his 1968 book, *The Rejuvenation Strategy.* Generally, Dr. Kiveloff says, it takes 6 to 8 weeks to produce a significant drop in high blood pressure, with long-term benefits growing over time.

Although it is possible to use Dr. Kiveloff's method to achieve good results without making other significant changes to your lifestyle, the information that follows will dramatically increase its effectiveness.

MUST READ—NOW!

Before you read the following Seven Golden Keys to lower blood pressure naturally, safely, and permanently, *please note that these suggestions DO NOT replace the advice of your medical doctor*. If you are taking medication at the present time, under no circumstances are you to stop taking it without your doctor's instructions. Also, feel free to share this entire chapter with your doctor. I assure you there is not a single word presented here that would contradict his or her medical advice.

SEVEN GOLDEN KEYS TO LOWER BLOOD PRESSURE NATURALLY, SAFELY, AND PERMANENTLY

1. Practice Dr. Kiveloff's full body Isometric Contraction exercise up to a dozen times per day. In addition, perform daily aerobic/cardio exercise (vigorous long walks are a great choice). Remember: physical *inactivity* increases the risk of obesity, diabetes, heart attack, and stroke. For this reason, daily exercise is a *must* for both prevention and treatment of high blood pressure.

2. Eat for health. As stated in the Nutrition Chapter, eat plenty of vegetables, fruits, 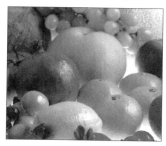 fiber, low-fat dairy products, and foods that are low in cholesterol. It is also important to reduce salt to a minimum or eliminate it entirely from your diet. Why? Because it contributes to high blood pressure due to increased fluid retention in the body. It has also been proven that a diet high in potassium, magnesium, and calcium (found in abundance in vegetables and fruit and low-fat dairy products) is very beneficial in both lowering and normalizing blood pressure.

3. If you are overweight, lose weight by following suggestions 1 & 2 above, until you are the ideal weight for your somatotype.

4. If you are a smoker, *quit*. With all the information available about the dangers of smoking, this seems to be a "no brainer," but consider that smoking 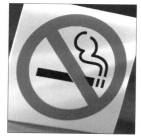 increases stress on the heart and arteries, which in turn increases the risk for a stroke and a cardiac event. It also contributes to elevated cholesterol and dramatically increases your risk for just about every known cancer. Bottom line: if you smoke, you need to quit...no brainer or not.

5. Avoid excess alcoholic consumption. Yes, I know there are studies that indicate a certain amount of wine can be beneficial to the heart and arteries. But there are people who take that information and use it as an excuse to drink more than they should. And even though there is scientific research that supports minimal alcoholic consump-

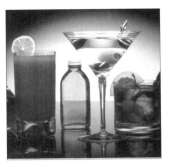

tion as being beneficial to health, there are also thousands of studies proving that excessive consumption of alcohol has devastating effects on one's health, including an elevation in blood pressure. Bottom line: if you drink, keep it to a minimum.

6. Avoid excess caffeine consumption. Once again, it is true that a certain amount of caffeine may be beneficial. But there is more than ample scientific evidence to prove that excess caffeine can have a devastating impact on one's health, including elevations in blood pressure and causing a host of chronic conditions, such as insomnia, heart palpitations, headaches, and nervousness (to name just a few). Bottom line: avoid caffeine as much as possible.

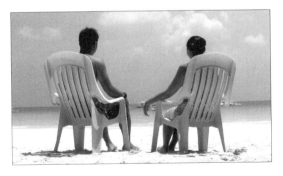

7. Relaxation and spiritual connection, or, in other words, "destressing." It is a fact that you can follow the first 6 recommendations to the letter and still be hypertensive. Why? Because emotional stress can literally eat you alive. Emotional stress can release hormones that elevate blood pressure and cause a wide range of physical problems. For that reason I want to recommend that you take time to intentionally relax.

I also recommend that you embark upon a spiritual quest and ask God to walk with you and direct your path. Don't get me wrong. I'm not trying to shove any brand of religion on you. But I am stating a fact. Just as Alcoholics Anonymous regards turning to a higher power (God) for help and direction as essential to one's recovery from alcohol addiction, so you need to ask God to help you with the personal issues in your life. If you are harboring anger, animosity, resentment, and unforgiveness toward others or yourself, you are carrying an emotional load 24/7 that is stressing you out and bound to have severe physiological consequences. This alone can place a tremendous strain on your emotions and consequently elevate your blood pressure. What to do? Turn to God, learn to forgive and let go of the past, and strive to live a life of compassion and forgiveness. If you do that, you will not only go a long way toward destressing your life and becoming a much happier person, you will help make the world a better place. To help you learn to forgive, memorize this quote from Longfellow: "If we could read the secret history of our enemies, we should find in each life sorrow and suffering enough to disarm all hostility."

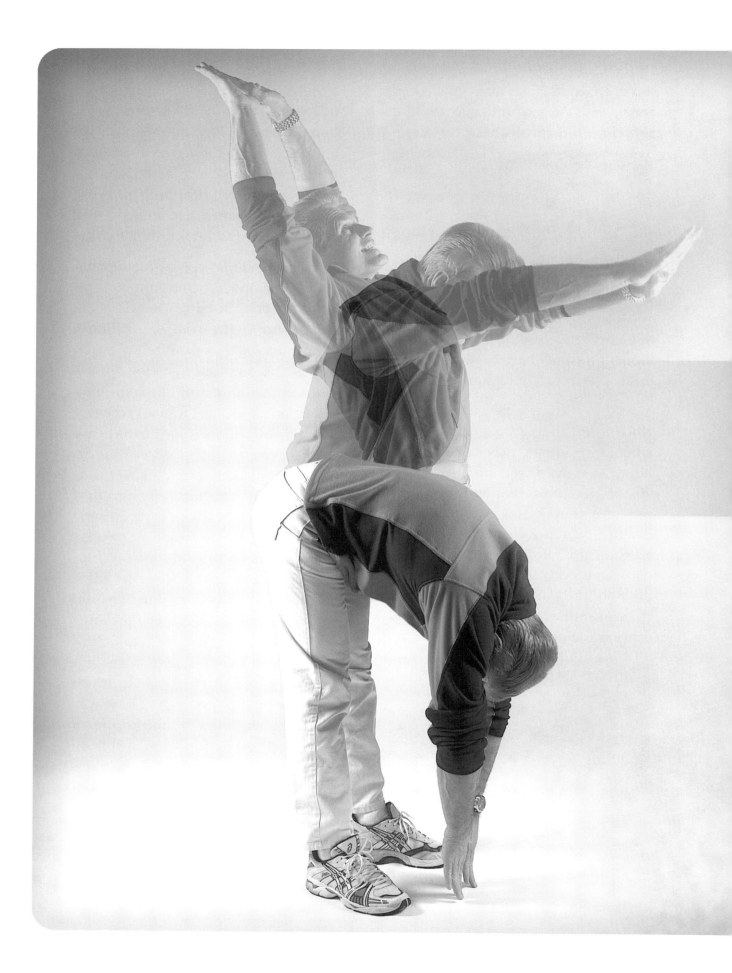

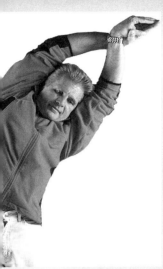
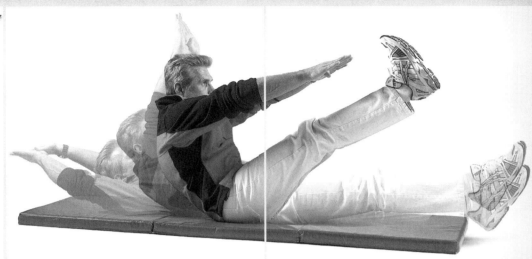

CHAPTER SIX

THE **MAGNIFICENT SEVEN**

Warming Up the Right Way

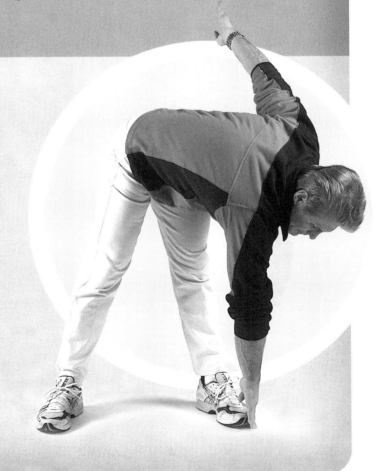

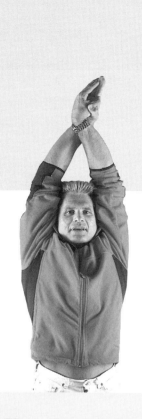

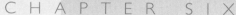

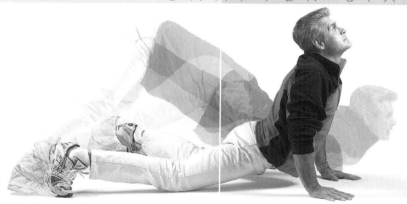

THE **MAGNIFICENT SEVEN**

Warming Up the Right Way

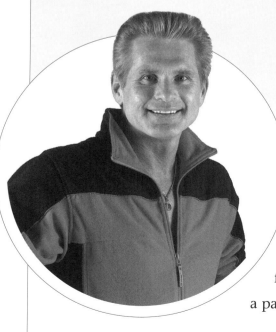

The Magnificent Seven are the ultimate warm-up exercises to help you achieve the most strength and benefit from your practice of Isometric Contraction. I have selected the seven exercises that have proven to be the best for stretching all the joints, tendons, ligaments, and muscles of the body, thus keeping them strong, flexible, and young. These movements will also slenderize the waistline very quickly. In fact, don't be surprised if you lose two or three inches from your waistline when you make the Magnificent Seven a part of your daily training. Here's why.

Although most people exercise in order to possess a handsome physique or figure, many people, particularly those who are older, want to regain the bodily proportion of their youth. By neglecting their health, they usually do not feel well, and their primary interest is to improve their health and appearance, which go hand in hand with physical development. They realize these are necessities in the building of a successful, happy, and vibrant life.

The fact is that we grow old when our joints, muscles, and arteries get stiff. To keep young and vibrant, it is necessary to exercise these joints, tendons, ligaments, muscles, and their attachments through a full range of motion. We must also increase our respiration and enhance our circulation with a pure bloodstream to keep our organs and glands young and efficient as well as to keep the arteries flexible and resilient and to keep the muscles working. The truth is we cannot be strong or active, cannot have energy and endurance, and cannot have good health unless we have strong and efficient internal organs, which are largely the result of performing exercises that involve the midsection (although good nutrition is important and does play a part of it).

The Magnificent Seven are designed to accomplish all these goals. These exercises strengthen your body *inside* as well as outside. The internal exercises strengthen and massage *all* the organs of the midsection, thus improving digestion, assimilation, and elimination. Remember, all movements of the body, internal and external, are muscular, and the more muscles you move, the more organs and glands are strengthened and their actions normalized. These are the motors of your body, and your life depends upon their efficiency.

Through the practice of the Magnificent Seven, you will gradually develop the ability to work without fatigue, to play harder, to enjoy meals more, and to not worry about internal discomfort or constipation. The gradual improvement of the organs and glandular functions makes it possible to walk and run farther and to extend yourself physically and mentally. You will build health, slenderize the waistline, improve your appearance, produce a maximum of flexibility and suppleness, and prepare your body to extend itself in the practice of the Isometric exercises that will greatly enhance both your strength and physique.

So now, let's warm up with the Magnificent Seven.

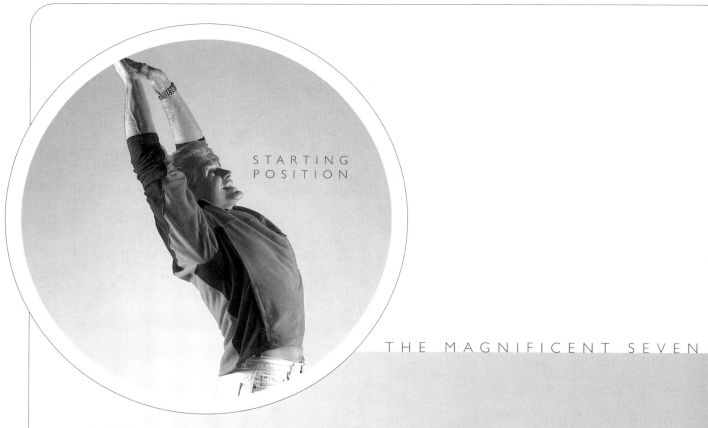

STARTING POSITION

EXERCISE #1
Forward Bend

This is a very simple exercise that stretches and activates the vital sections of the body and will help keep you young.

Stand with your feet a comfortable distance apart and raise both your arms straight over your head and bend well back from the small of your back. Then bend forward, endeavoring to touch the floor between your feet with both hands while keeping your legs as straight as possible. Practice this exercise steadily, exhaling as you touch the floor, inhaling as your arms are raised above your head. Start with 6 complete movements, then on every third day increase the repetitions by 1 until you are performing 12 repetitions for warm-up purposes and up to 36 to enhance athletic fitness and trim the waistline.

This exercise imparts increased flexibility to the muscles and the spine and activates the nerve centers of the lower back, which is the vital section of the body. It stretches the tendons and muscles of this region, the sacrum, the sacroiliac, and the hips. It promotes youth and increased elasticity in the involved parts of the body and builds endurance in walking and running.

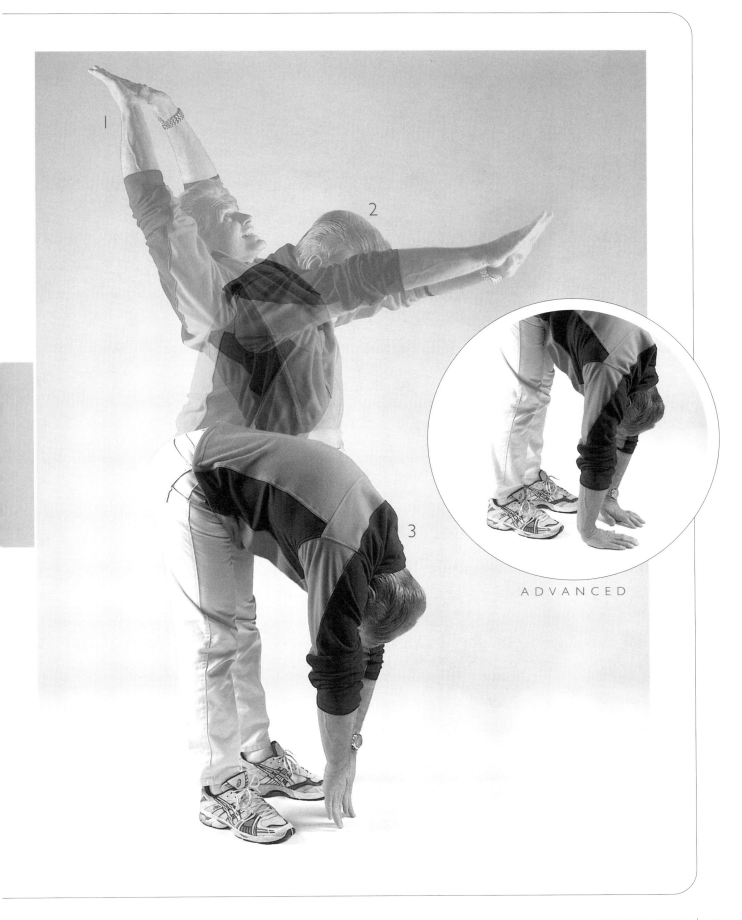

1

2

3

ADVANCED

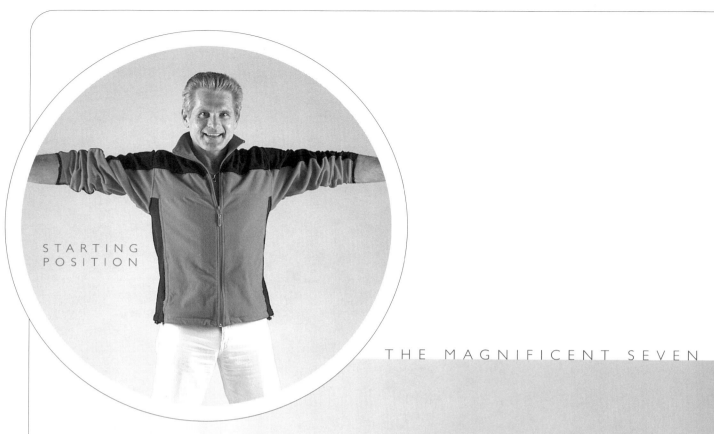

STARTING
POSITION

EXERCISE #2
Up, Over, and Down

In his bestselling *The Golden Keys to Internal Physical Fitness,* Paul Bragg called this exercise "The One, the Only Perfect Exercise—This Is It—the Best!" Why? Because it stretches nearly every one of the 600 muscles in the body.

Stand with your feet shoulder-width apart or slightly wider, arms extended straight from your sides and forming a straight line across your shoulders. Swing your right arm up and overhead counterclockwise and continue down across the body while bending from the waist with your knees stiff and touch (or try to touch) your left big toe (see photo). You may not make it the first time, but stretch down as far as you can. When your back and hips become more supple, you will easily touch your left big toe. Then reverse direction, swinging your arm overhead fast but under control and bend backward from the waist. All this should be one continuous movement.

Now repeat with your left arm, stretching up, over, and down to the right big toe. While performing this exercise, suck in and blow out air forcefully, exhaling while touching the big toe and inhaling while changing sides. Do this exercise 6 times to each side (12 repetitions total)

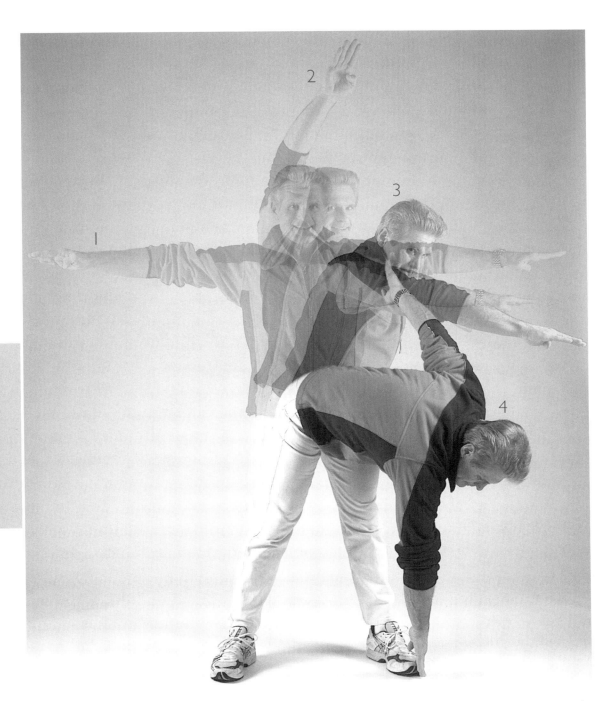

and add 1 repetition every 3 days until you are performing 12 repetitions to each side for a total of 24 repetitions as a warm-up. For enhanced athletic fitness and fat loss, perform up to 36 repetitions to each side.

This superb exercise removes external and internal fat from the entire midsection (front, back, and sides), activates the internal organs and glands, improves all the processes of digestion and elimination, imparts exceptional suppleness and a high level of strength to the body parts involved.

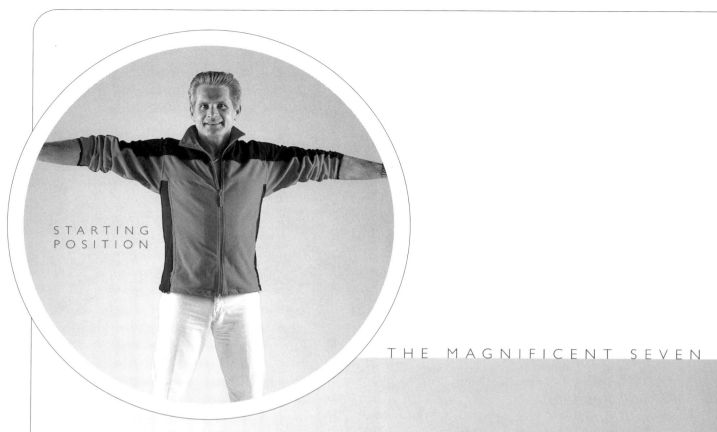

STARTING
POSITION

EXERCISE #3
Side-to-Side Twist

This is a simple but highly effective exercise to reduce fat inside and outside the midsection, to develop the strength of the muscles, and to keep the vertebrae loose and flexible.

Assume the position shown with your arms fully extended to the sides as in the previous exercise, forming a straight line across the shoulders. Keeping your arms directly opposite of each other as if held in place by a long pole parsed across the back of the neck and shoulders, swing your arms and shoulders in unison. Twist one direction and then the other until the line of your arms at the extreme tension of the swing is as nearly as possible at right angles to the starting position and your feet. The greatest flexibility will be found in the upper region of the spine, allowing a slight flexing of each section of the vertebrae and giving an aggregate twist that will increase with continual practice. Remember: your shoulders must swing with your arms or the movement has little value. The object is to make the twist with your upper body, so your hips should keep their natural position facing forward during the exercise and not swing side to side with your arms and shoulders. Start with 6 repetitions in each direction and add 1 repetition every 3 workouts until you are performing 12 repetitions in each direction for warm-up purposes. If you desire enhanced athletic strength and flexibility, you may work up to 36 repetitions in each direction.

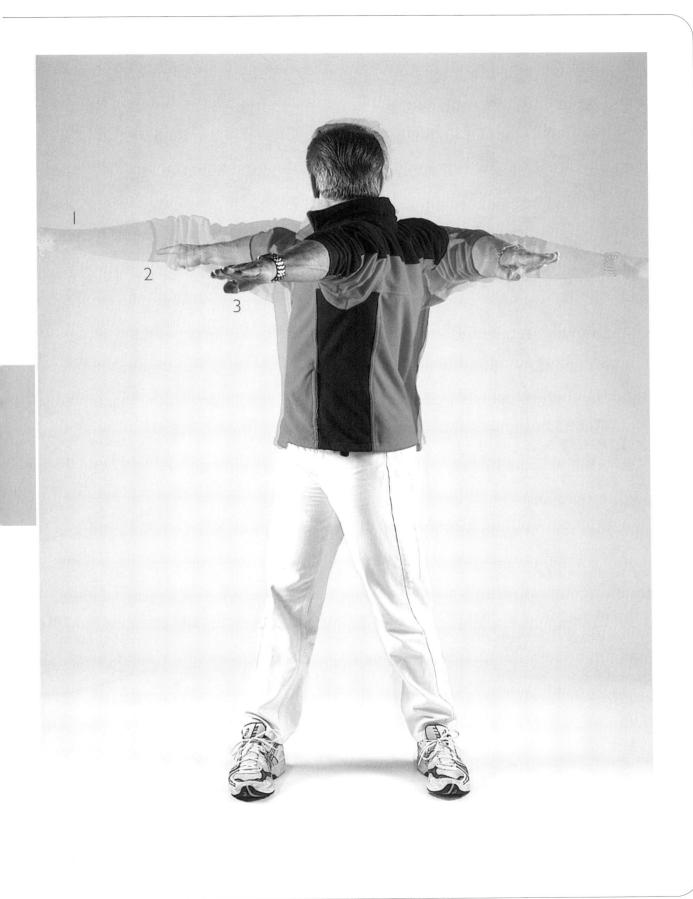

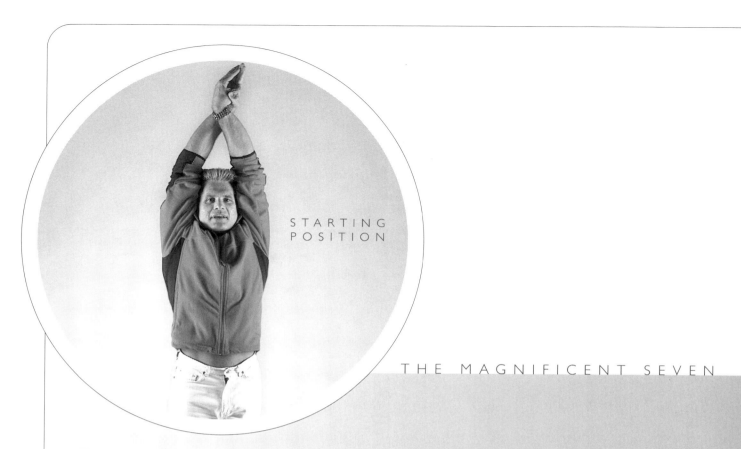

STARTING
POSITION

EXERCISE #4

Torso Circle

Stand with your heels together and raise your arms straight over your head in a reverse hand-clasp as shown. Your arms are kept straight with your upper arms tight to your ears throughout this movement. Moving only from the waist, make a large enough circular movement so that you can feel the tension in the muscles of your lower back, sides, and the front abdomen as you turn or twist. The "Torso Circle" strengthens the muscles of your sides, abdomen, and back and reduces weight around the waist both inside and out, and it has a stimulating effect on all the internal organs. For warm-up purposes, begin with 6 repetitions in each direction and increase by 1 every 3 workouts until you are performing 12 in each direction for a total of 24 repetitions. Those who want to dramatically reduce the size of their waistline may wish to work up to 36 repetitions in each direction. You'll soon discover that this exercise hits the entire midsection—front, back, and sides—as no other exercise does.

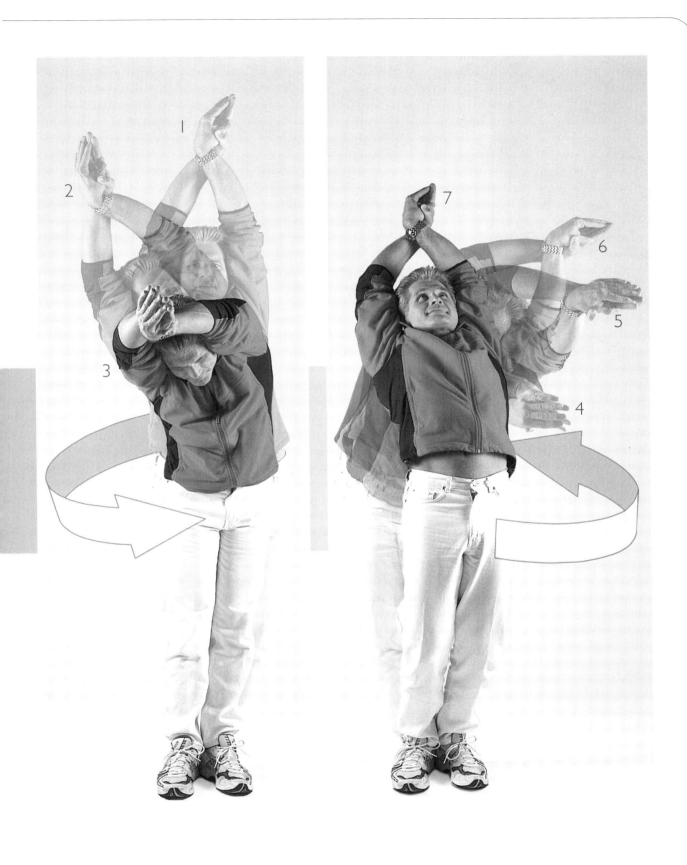

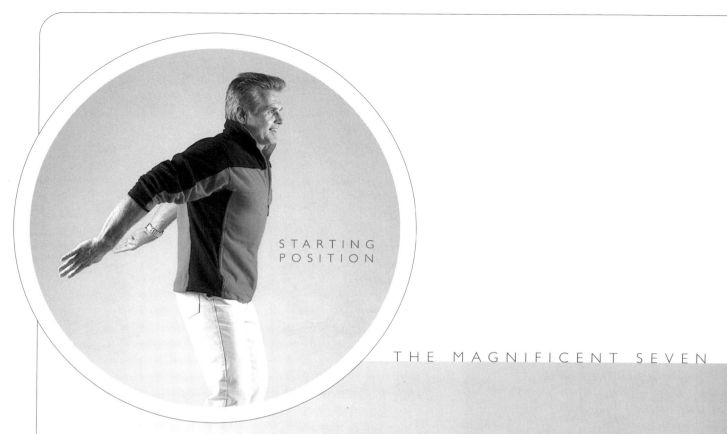

STARTING
POSITION

EXERCISE #5

Tiger Bend Squat

This exercise is of tremendous value in perfecting poise, balance, and suppleness of the entire body while dramatically enhancing leg strength.

Assume a standing position as shown with your hands at your sides. Draw your arms backward until your hands are about 18" from the vertical line of your body. Lower your body into the low deep knee bend position. As your body descends, bring your arms forward and by continuing their swing the balance of your body will be easier to maintain while bending and rising. This exercise not only strengthens the legs and hips in a dramatic way but can also enhance cardio endurance to a tremendous extent when performed in sets of 50 to 100 repetitions or more. However, for warm-up purposes, start with 6 repetitions and add 1 repetition every 3 workouts until you are practicing 12 to 36 repetitions on a consistent basis. I personally believe the Tiger Bend Squat and the Tiger Bend Push-up are two of the best full body dynamic exercises in the entire realm of physical culture.

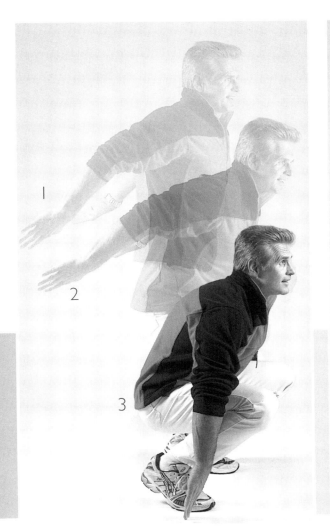

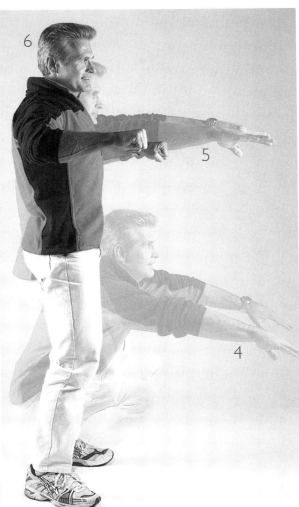

1

2

3

4

5

6

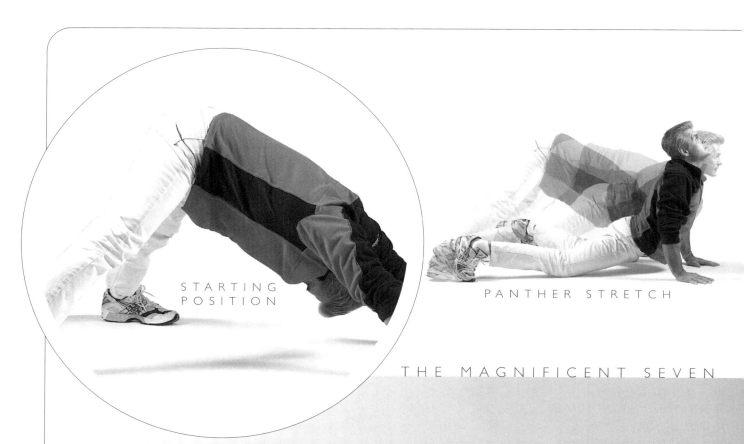

STARTING POSITION

PANTHER STRETCH

EXERCISE #6
Tiger Stretch Push-up

This may be the oldest exercise known to man. It has been practiced in the Middle East, India, and the Orient for thousands of years. Once you see it performed, it is obvious why it is called the Tiger Stretch Push-up, as it virtually duplicates the movement of large jungle cats. Although they are caged in small pens at the zoo or circus, they are as amazingly strong and fit in captivity as they would be in the wild. Pacing back and forth and stretching their muscles under tension (identical to this exercise) are their only exercises. So the results are obvious.

The movement of this exercise is ideal for strengthening and slenderizing the midsection and improves the action of all internal organs and glands. Perhaps more importantly, it stretches and strengthens all the muscles, tendons, and ligaments of the entire body from neck to toes on both sides of the body as it imparts youth and flexibility of movement.

Start this movement in the position as shown in photo 1, hands on the floor, shoulder-width apart, and your head tucked in looking directly at your feet. Your feet are a little wider than shoulder-width apart. Your legs and back are straight, and your butt is the highest point of the body. Next, bend your elbows while descending in a smooth circular arc as shown in photos 2–4.

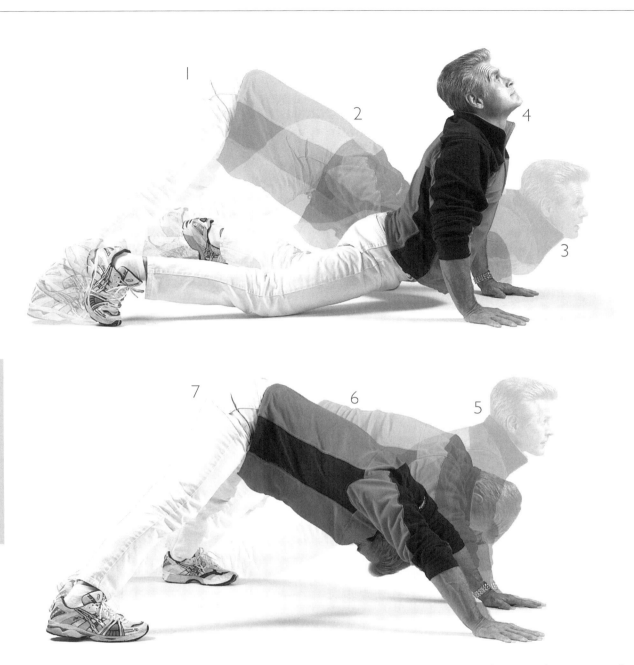

Almost brush your chest and upper body to the floor as you continue the circular range of motion until your arms are straight, your back is flexed, and your hips are almost touching the floor. At the top of the movement, stretch your neck back and look up at the ceiling while consciously flexing your triceps and inhaling (see photo 4). At this point, return to the starting position by raising your hips and buttocks while simultaneously pushing back with straight arms (photo 5–6), causing a complete articulation of the shoulder joints. Arrive at the starting position (photo 7) and continue. Start with 6 repetitions and gradually add repetitions as you are able. No need to perform more than 12 repetitions for warm-up purposes, but those who want to dramatically enhance their athletic performance may desire to perform 36 or more.

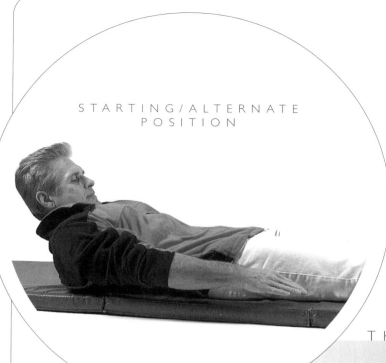

THE MAGNIFICENT SEVEN

EXERCISE #7
The Abdominal Double Curl

This exercise was recommended by Dr. Frank Rudolph Young (page 220) as the ultimate exercise for sculpted abs and enhanced sexual vigor.

Begin flat on your back on a soft surface. As you inhale, lift your head and shoulders up and forward (photo 2) followed by straight legs to a point of momentary balance on your tailbone at the top of the inhale and movement, so that you balance like a "v." Exhaling down, place your heels on the floor, then uncurl the upper body until your head rests on the floor. Remember: your head is the first part of your body to move up and the last to relax down. Start with 6 repetitions and add 1 repetition every 3 workouts until you are performing 12 repetitions for warm-up purposes and work up to 36 for ab sculpting. You will soon discover that Dr. Young knew what he was talking about when outlining the benefits of this superb exercise.

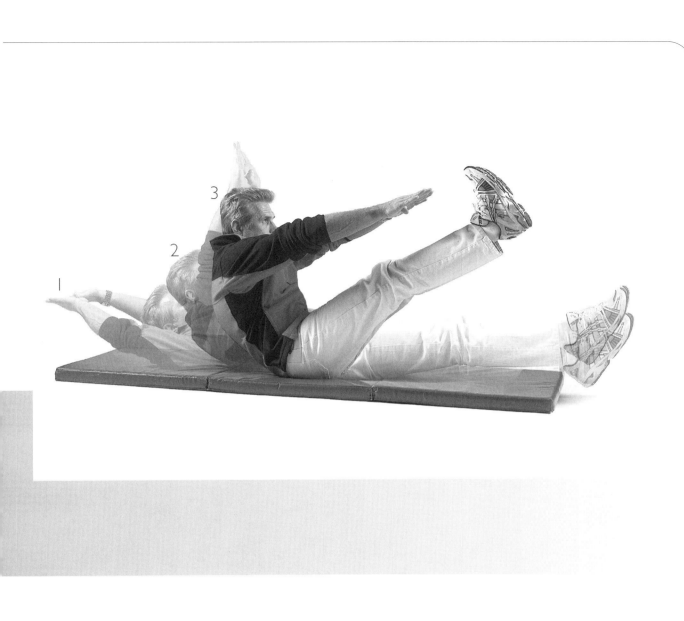

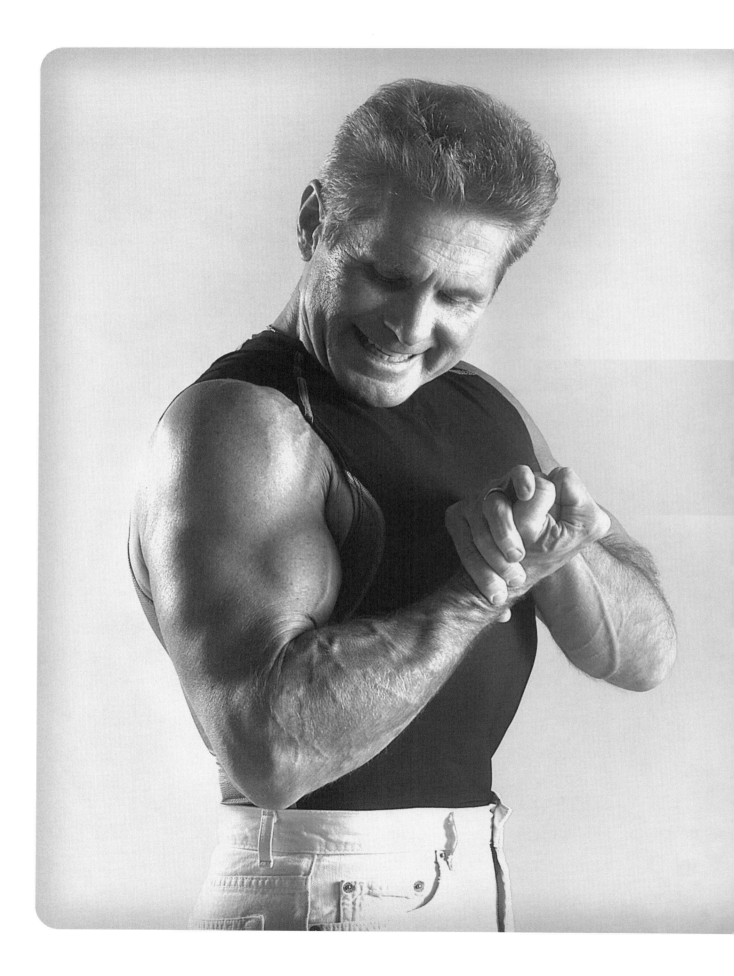

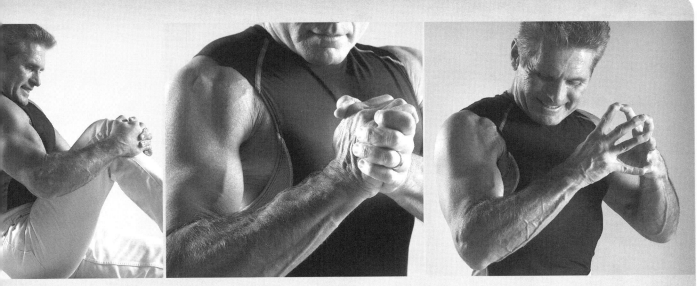

CHAPTER SEVEN

CLASSIC ISOMETRICS *for a* POWERFUL PHYSIQUE

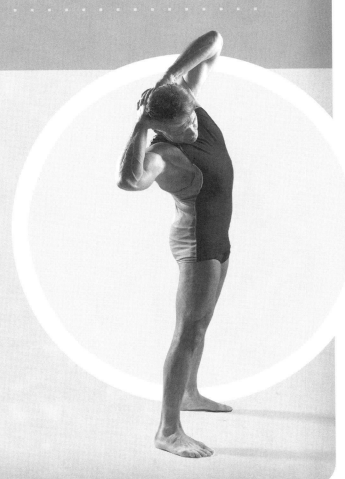

DEEP BREATHING ALONE
has made many a sick man well
and many a weak man STRONG.

—Farmer Burns

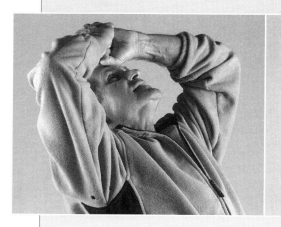

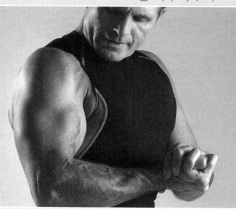

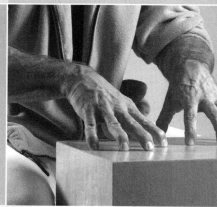

CLASSIC ISOMETRICS *for a* POWERFUL PHYSIQUE

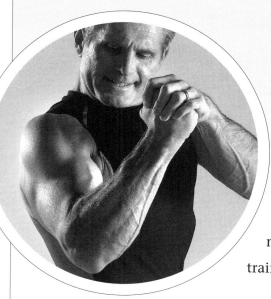

Now that you have read the first six chapters of *The Isometric Power Revolution*, I hope that you are excited about taking the information and knowledge that you have just gained and are ready to turn it into personal wisdom by applying these techniques and methods specifically to your own body's needs. Then and only then will these master methods become a part of your personal body wisdom and training philosophy.

However, before I go any further, I want to address one pertinent issue that many people question because of the misinformation about exercise that is perpetuated by equipment manufacturers whose primary goal is monetary gain. That issue is whether or not it is really possible to achieve superior results and a super state of physical manhood without relying on anything outside of yourself, particularly, the equipment we all see advertised in those ubiquitous exercise machine infomercials that are playing 24/7 on television stations everywhere. And the answer to that question is a very affirmative YES!

In fact, the only way one can achieve a super state of complete mind/body and muscular self-mastery is through the applicatioin of methods that unite mind and body as one, such as those that are presented here. But there is another reason for becoming a master of our training methods and for not using methods that rely on equipment or that cause compression to the lower spine. And to explain it to you succinctly, I am once again turning to the writings of master physical culturist Tromp Van Diggelen and his autobiography *Worth While Journey*, published in 1955. On pages 248 and 249, Van Diggelen stated the following, with which I completely agree.

"No organ of the body can function properly without an adequate nerve stimulus. The nerves of the body need blood in the same manner that the root of a plant needs water. It will be clear to you now that the body cannot be really healthy without a vigorous spinal blood circulation. One of my most important principles is that, by the practice of firm contraction and complete relaxation, without the use of apparatus, weights or rubber exercises, the best possible nutrition is obtained for the spinal muscles and the spinal cord.

Some systems employ machine-like movements of whole groups of muscles without training a man or woman to concentrate on individual muscles. It is the consciously controlled action of individual muscles which is so valuable in the conservation of energy and the building of a healthy mind and body."

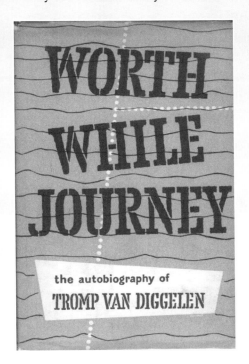

What Van Diggelen has stated in the above paragraphs is absolutely correct. When one achieves a superior state of physical/mental self-mastery so that he or she can positively contract or relax any given muscle group throughout the entire body at will and do so without relying on any form of apparatus outside of the body, one has reached a super state of body awareness and mind/muscle mastery that can be achieved in no other way. Simply put, the nerve impulses to all of the muscles, glands, and various tissues throughout the entire body will be greatly enhanced and not impeded in any way. This in turn will keep you younger far longer than any other method you could possibly use because you are doing nothing to cause a breakdown anywhere within the skeletal system.

As a result, you *will* look great, you *will* feel great, and you *will* become a *great deal stronger* if you follow the methods we teach. C'mon, you already got a taste of it when you performed the Isometric Deep Breathing Exercise in Chapter 1. That alone will strengthen you in a significant way. Remember what Farmer Burns said? Write it down and memorize it. "Deep breathing alone has made many a sick man well and many a weak man strong." And it is absolutely true.

You've also seen evidence of what will happen to your physique and body as a result of following these methods from the facts presented in Chapter 2—A Concise History of Isometric Contraction. (And, no, you don't have to bite through nails and chains.) So now in Chapter 7, we're going to teach you how to strengthen and sculpt every muscle in your entire body from your neck to your toes with Classic Isometric Contraction.

However, before I teach you what to do, I must address a ridiculous excuse that many people use for not getting the best out of themselves, for not reaching their potential or achieving the greatness that God placed in them. What excuse am I referring to? In a word: *genetics*.

DEEP BREATHING ALONE
has made many a sick man well
and many a weak man STRONG.

—Farmer Burns

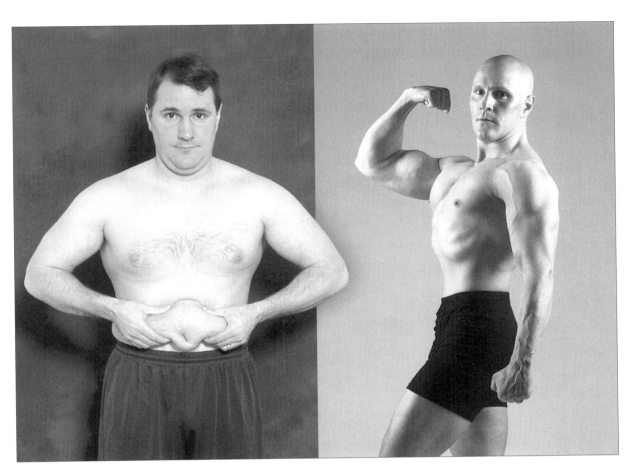

GENETICS: THE MYTH THAT HOLDS SOME PEOPLE BACK

(Don't fall for it.)

Take a look at these contrasting photos. Would you believe that the man on the left is, in fact, the man on the right, and that the photos were taken less than one year apart? Would you even dream that the man on the left could become the man on the right? Well, it's true. They're the same man. His name is Dr. Neal Eslinger, and he has become a very close personal friend of mine. He personifies everything we teach at Bronze Bow.

How did Dr. Neal transform himself from picture A to picture B in less than a year?

First, by not allowing himself to have any stupid excuses that would hold him back. He would be the first to tell you to not believe the "genetics excuse"—that we are genetically stuck with our bodies, and that we can't do a thing about it. He is quick to point out that we all have the same muscle groups. All can be strengthened through proper exercise and good nutrition, and all can be wasted through lack of exercise and bad nutrition. He had a choice to make regarding what he was going to do with his body, and he obviously made the right one. We are all free to make the right choice.

Let me tell you a little about him. Dr. Neal Eslinger has a thriving chiropractic practice. He chose our methods because he wanted to discover for himself the best, most positive methods to share with his clients in order to help them rehabilitate old injuries. (Let's face it, instead of doing the smart thing and visiting a chiropractor as a part of a lifelong health and youthfuless program, most people wait until they are hurting.) He also wanted to help his clients prevent new injuries from happening while he helped them become strong and fit. So in order to prove the validity of our methods, Dr. Eslinger first tested our methods on himself, thereby transforming himself into the epitome of manly strength, fitness, and physique. He accomplished what you see without relying on weights or equipment of any kind.

That's why I asked Dr. Eslinger to pose for many of the exercise photos in this book. Who better than a man who has proven the worth of these methods on himself, and a man who uses them with his clients?

CLASSIC ISOMETRIC CONTRACTION

In this first section on strength enhancement and physique development, we will use Classic Isometric Contraction (CIC). You already know what I mean by this term from reading Chapter 2. (If you didn't read Chapter 2, you're cheating yourself.) By CIC, I'm referring to Isometrics where we work against an immovable force or object and do so at several positions or angles within any range of movement. In this case the immovable force is supplied by another group of muscles.

CIC is a key component for developing the super human strength that both Alexander Zass and The Mighty Atom displayed. The essential factor to this form of Isometric Contraction is that it builds strength from the inside out rather than the outside in. It accomplishes this by first strengthening tendons and ligaments and stabilizing the joints, and *then* strengthening the muscles. This type of training causes the muscles to become very dense and firm to the touch.

CIC also causes the body to "heat up" very quickly. Seriously, in just 5 minutes of utilizing intense CICs you can and will be drenched in sweat. This is also why it causes such dramatic increases in muscular definition. Why? Because as the body "heats up" and you combine Isometrics with deep breathing, it's like incinerating body fat on the hurry-up. I have thousands of students and friends around the world who will attest to this. In fact, usually within two weeks, most people experience a dramatic improvement in muscular definition.

How is this possible? Here's at least one concrete reason: because Isometrics work the muscles in the most direct way possible with the utmost of intensity.

Plus, CIC allows you to work the muscles far more safely than any other method. Why? Because the load on any given muscle at any given angle is gradually increased for 3 to 4 seconds until peak contraction is achieved, maintained for 7 to 12 seconds at peak intensity, and then slowly released for another 3 to 4 seconds. There is no jerking or "cheating" as is common with weight training. And there's no reliance on amplified gravity (weight) to create the contraction. Hence, it does not cause a sudden and intense pull at the juncture of muscles and tendons, and it does not compress the lower spine. Not only that, but with CIC the tendons become phenomenally strong, unlike some exercise methods where the muscles become far stronger than the tendons. When that happens, injury is almost guaranteed.

So let's take a serious look at the muscle structures of the body and see why they should be developed and why Isometrics is the best way to strengthen them.

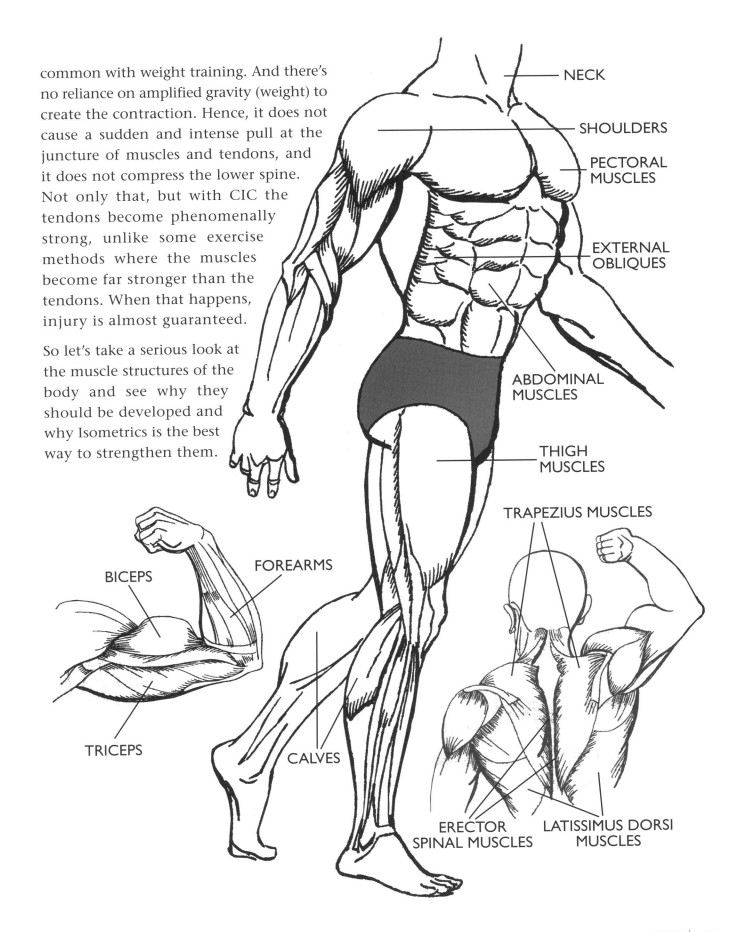

NECK

SHOULDERS

PECTORAL MUSCLES

EXTERNAL OBLIQUES

ABDOMINAL MUSCLES

THIGH MUSCLES

TRAPEZIUS MUSCLES

BICEPS

FOREARMS

TRICEPS

CALVES

ERECTOR SPINAL MUSCLES

LATISSIMUS DORSI MUSCLES

IMPORTANT MUSCLES OF THE BODY

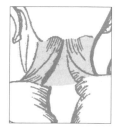

1. The Neck

One of the most important muscle groups in the entire body is the neck. Yet most fitness programs don't even mention the neck—not even a whisper in passing. So, friends, here's the only time you'll read me saying anything negative about my competitors. If a so-called, self-professed expert has you working only the muscles that show, trust me, he or she is no expert (except in his or her own mind).

Think about it. Your neck supports the entire weight of your head. It has both a muscular and joint structure that allows you to turn 180° from side to side and to swivel a full 360°. It houses the top of the entire spinal column, and if it gets broken due to a car accident or a sport injury, you can be paralyzed instantly from the neck down for life. In fact, that's exactly what happened to actor Christopher Reeve, who played Super Man. He broke his neck after being thrown from his horse, and his entire body was paralyzed until the day he died.

My point is this: it is foolish to develop only the muscles that show while a vital muscle structure such as the neck is left weak and undeveloped, especially if you could prevent the damage that comes from an accident that leaves you paralyzed for life. Especially when in less than 5 minutes a day you could have a superbly developed neck by following my neck development program. There is a saying that "a chain is only as strong as its weakest link." It's true, and if a fitness program doesn't develop the neck first, this program's weak link is exposed and not worth doing.

You will find a complete neck developing program beginning on page 144.

2. Trapezius Muscles

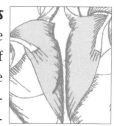

On both sides of the shoulders at the base of the neck on top of the shoulders are the trapezius muscles. Strong, well-developed trapezius muscles help keep the shoulders in their proper place and enhance one's posture. But in addition to good posture, developing these muscles also helps competitors in all contact sports to remain injury free.

If you have weak trapezius muscles, you will be round-shouldered and have a weak neck. Both the neck and trapezius development exercises found on pages 144–153 will correct this condition. In fact, all neck exercises also develop the trapezius.

3. Shoulders

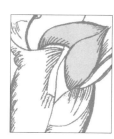

Broad, powerful shoulders are envied by men and admired by women. They not only enhance a man's appearance but also enhance a man's ability in virtually every contact sport from boxing, wrestling, and every martial art to tennis, golf, football, baseball, basketball, and hockey. To build the strength of your shoulders, perform the exercises on pages 154–161.

4. Pectoral Muscles

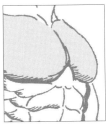

The function of the pectoral muscles is to move the arms forward, downward, and across the chest. These muscles, which cover the chest, enhance the appearance of one's physique when fully developed and greatly enhance one's ability in all contact and racquet sports. The pectorals respond very quickly to CIC, especially when combined with various types of push-ups. The exercises for pectoral development are found on pages 180–185.

5. Latissimus Dorsi Muscles

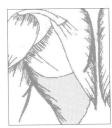

The latissimus dorsi muscles are the large fanned-shaped muscles of the upper back, beginning at the armpits and extending all the way to the waistline. In fact, it was these muscles that Jean Valjean had developed through his consistant use of Isometric Contraction as found on page 90 of *Les Misérables* ("A full course of mysterious statics") that tipped off Inspector Javert as to who Valjean really was. If you want to know more, read Victor Hugo's *Les Misérables*.

The function of the latissimus dorsi muscles is to lower the arms and move them backward. In men who have wide shoulders and small waists, these muscles give a very distinctive V-shaped when

fully developed. For obvious reasons, gymnasts and swimmers usually have beautifully shaped latissimus dorsi muscles. The CIC exercises found on pages 186–189 will quickly develop these muscles as well as enhance your ability to play many sports.

If you wish to test the strength of your "lats," here's an easy method: see how many times you can "chin the bar," then perform CICs exclusively for 30 days and retest yourself. Don't be surprised if your improvement is 100 percent. It happened for my friend Andrew McDuffy, who went from 4 reps to 10 reps as a result of doing what we teach. So if someone tries to tell you these exercises won't work, tell them to stick it in their ear.

6. Erector Spinal Muscles

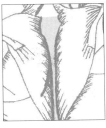

The erector spinal muscles resemble two large steel cables that run along both sides of the spinal column. They may not look nearly as impressive as the latissimus dorsi muscles, but in terms of function, they are far more vital because they support the spine and protect the vertebrae and spinal cord itself. It is essential to keep these muscles strong and well developed if one wishes to avoid lower back pain and lumbago that are suffered by millions of Americans.

Many exercises that rely on heavy weights, such as dead lifts, good mornings, and squats, will certainly develop the erector spinal muscles, but the amplified gravitational force pulling down will literally destroy the discs that separate and cushion the vertebrae, which is why heavy weightlifting often has disastrous consequences. The good news is that if you follow the CIC protocols presented in this program, you can develop every bit as much strength or more without *any* of the negative side effects.

REMEMBER: strength is essential to succeed in all contact sports from martial arts to rugby and everything in between, but it's how you achieve great strength that makes all the difference in the world. CICs will help you accomplish that goal far more safely than any other method, especially when it comes to developing the erector spinal muscles. The exercises described on pages 190–193 will develop these muscles and protect you from injury.

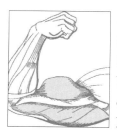

7. Biceps and Triceps

Everyone would like to have beautifully developed biceps and triceps. Some desire it just because it looks great, and others because it dramatically enhances their sports performance, whether it's baseball, basketball, football, racquet sports, golf, or martial arts. Though most people are more concerned about their biceps, the truth is that the biceps, which are flexors, need to be balanced by triceps development, which are extensors.

The biceps are located on the front of the upper arm and are responsible for pulling things toward you. For instance, chinning the bar pulls your body toward the bar and dramatically engages the biceps. The triceps, on the other hand, push things away or extend and push them away from a bent position until the arms are fully extended. In many sports, such as baseball, boxing, fencing, or gymnastics, it is critical that biceps and triceps be balanced in both strength and endurance in order to achieve mastery. No form of exercise allows one to work on strength and endurance deficiencies as well as CICs and to overcome weaknesses within any plane of motion.

You will find exercises for biceps and triceps development on pages 162–167. Whether you want functional athletes' strength or great looking arms, you will achieve both aims with these exercises.

8. Hands, Wrists, and Forearms

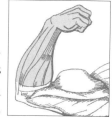

Developing the hands, wrists, and forearms is crucial for excelling in many sports, such as auto racing, archery, gymnastics, racquet sports, golf, baseball, and virtually all contact sports. You need a strong grip. But it's also essential for everyday life. Consider, for instance, a stubborn jar lid, or raking leaves, or doing yard work. You need strong hands, wrists, and forearms. The good news is that Isometrics will strengthen and develop the tendons, ligaments, and muscles faster than any other method.

Remember the ancient archers from Chapter 2? Point made. You'll find excellent exercises for hands, wrists, and forearms beginning on page 168–179.

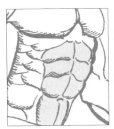

9. Abdominal Muscles

In recent years, no muscle group has received as much attention in books, magazines, and infomercials as has the abdominal muscles. From a health perspective, I couldn't agree more. Strong, well-defined abdominals will help to maintain youthfulness and vigor as nothing else will for both men and women. If fact, I'll go on record as saying the abdominals are the most important muscle structure of the entire body to develop, whether you are an athlete or not. This is because the function of every gland and organ is enhanced when one has developed powerful abdominal muscles. They aid both digestion and elimination.

If you do nothing other than follow the exercises for complete abdominal development on pages 196–199, it will repay you many times your investment in health, strength, and vibrancy.

10. External Oblique Muscles

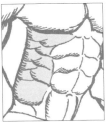

These are the muscles on both sides of the abdomen and lower back. When well developed, these muscles stabilize the entire upper body structure and add great strength and power to all twisting movements, whether you're belting home runs, fighting for the heavyweight championship, or lifting your little boy or girl from a car seat. The point is, these muscles are important, and they need to be strengthened and developed along with your abdominals. You will notice that the external obliques are in both ab-specific programs. For complete development, turn to pages 194–195.

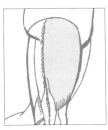

11. Thigh and Hip Muscles

The thighs and hips are the largest and most powerful muscles in the body. Muscular, athletic legs are not only pleasing to look at but are also a necessity. These muscles literally carry us through life and will keep us years younger and stronger than our contemporaries when we develop them and keep them strong and fit.

For all sports and athletics, strong legs are an obvious necessity. In boxing, baseball, basketball, tennis, the martial arts, track, and football, the loss of strength, endurance, and stamina will end a career in a hurry. But it need not be so. For example, when I was a kid the light heavyweight champion of the world, Archie Moore, was defending his title when he was well past 50 years of age, and the reason he could was because of his extraordinary strength and conditioning. So if you want to stay young, strong, and virile for life, perform the exercises found on pages 200–211 and keep your thighs and hips strong for life.

12. Calves

The calves, together with the feet, are the foundation upon which your entire body stands, and as a foundation it should be

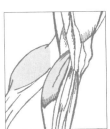

the strongest that you can possibly make it. Strengthening and shaping your calves will let you stand longer, walker farther, run faster, and jump higher than you ever thought possible.

CLASSIC ISOMETRIC CONTRACTION EXERCISES FOR HEALTH, STRENGTH, AND A SCULPTED PHYSIQUE

I learned the following series of CIC exercises to strengthen and sculpt every muscle in the entire body from your neck to your toes from my uncle Milo. Please note that absolutely no equipment other than a chair and wall is ever needed. Most of these exercises can be performed virtually anywhere—at home, at the office, in school, or riding on a bus or train. All of them will strengthen tendons and ligaments as well as muscles, producing strength that is truly functional.

All of the CIC exercises are *easy* to learn. *However,* that is the only *easy* thing about them. CICs can and will produce magnificent results, but they require a laser-like focus between your mind and your muscles and the ability to push yourself to maintain incredibly high levels of tension for 7 to 12 seconds in duration. Trust me: there is nothing *easy* about it. For *all* of them, the following seven rules apply.

THE SEVEN GOLDEN RULES OF ISOMETRIC POWER

I. All exercises using the right arm, right leg, or any muscle group on the right side of the body MUST also be repeated with the left arm, left leg, or the corresponding part on the left side of the body with equal intensity. *No Exceptions.* This will ensure symmetrical development.

2. With few exceptions, each CIC will be held at three angles within any given range of motion. These positions include:

A. Near full extension—the muscle in most stretched position.

B. Midway between full extension and peak contraction.

C. Peak contraction—the muscle is at its shortest, most contracted position.

NOTE: Theories abound about which position yields the greatest result. But the way I view it, why leave any room for doubt when you can exercise the muscle at all three angles? Only a lazy moron or couch potato would complain about the multi-angle approach.

3. When possible, especially as you are learning the exercises, perform the exercises in front of a mirror and wear as little clothing as possible. This accomplishes three goals. First, it helps you learn proper form when you compare your form to the form you see in the book photos. Second, it helps you comprehend how the muscles respond at various levels of contraction and intensity: "This is how it looks, and this is how it feels at this level of contraction." And, third, when you can see your muscles contracting, it becomes easier to focus and intensify your contractions.

4. The intensity of either pushing or pulling and the resistance to it must also be of equal intensity so that there is *no movement,* whether your muscles are being contracted at 30 or 70 percent or more of maximum strength. The level of contraction and opposing force must remain equal at all times.

5. Correct breathing procedure—there are three phases to each contraction.

- Slowly build contraction to peak intensity for 3 to 4 seconds while *deeply inhaling.*

- Upon reaching peak contraction, slowly start a controlled exhalation in order to maintain uniform intrathoraxic pressure. This is done by making an *f-f-f-f or s-s-s-s* sound as you exhale air slowly through closed teeth or lips. It should literally sound like air being released from a tire. This procedure should last from 7 to 12 seconds while maintaining great intensity during the contraction.

- Slowly release tension for 3 to 4 seconds while inhaling.

6. Relax completely between exercises by power breathing as deeply as possible for 7 to 10 repetitions while intentionally relaxing your muscles and making them as soft and supple as you possibly can. This will dramatically enhance results by oxygenating the working muscles with fresh oxygen-rich blood, which will make it possible for you to train with still greater intensity.

7. Follow the first six rules to the letter. Your success depends on it.

Now that you know the rules, let's get back to the rat killin'. We'll start at the neck and systematically work the entire muscle structure of the body right down to your calves.

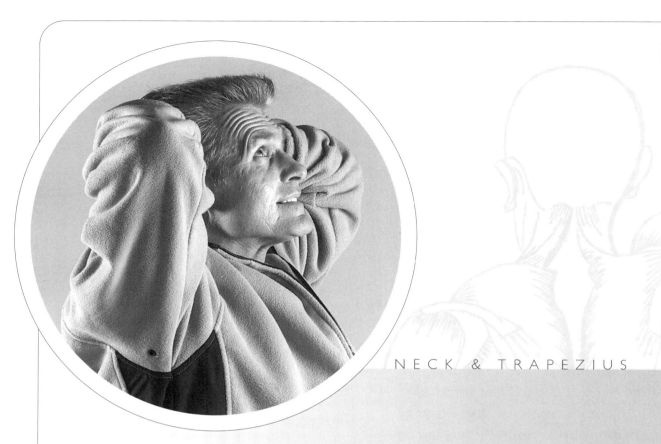

NECK EXERCISE #1
Reverse Neck Contraction

POSITION A: Stand erect with your feet about 12" apart. Clasp your hands behind your head and interlock your fingers with your chin tucked close to the chest as shown. Now push your head firmly up while resisting with your hands. Maintain an intense contraction 7 to 12 seconds while following correct breathing procedures. Relax.

POSITIONS B AND C: Repeat exercise following the same breathing procedures, relaxing and then moving to exercise #2.

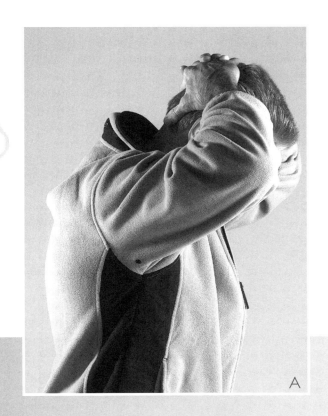

A

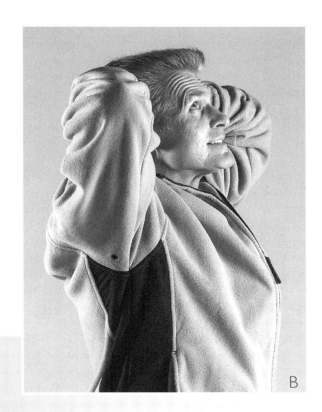

B

POSITIONS

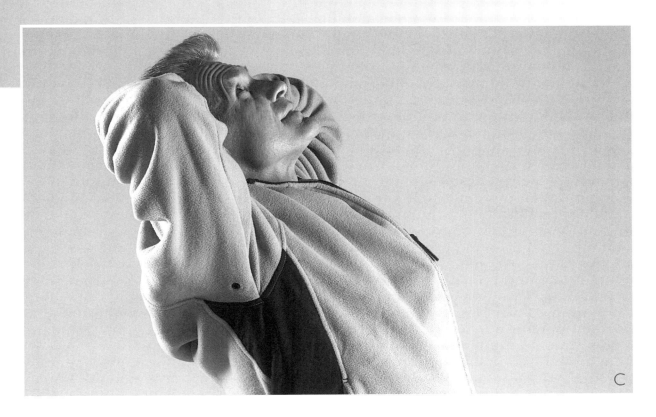

C

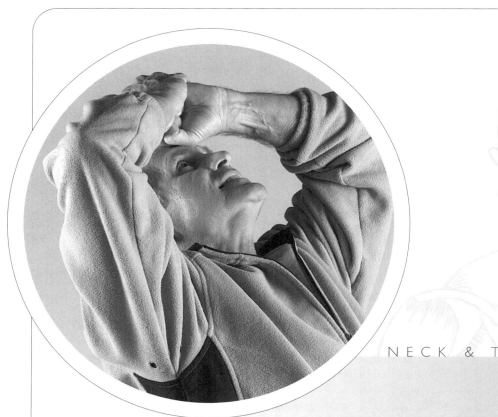

NECK EXERCISE #2
Forward Neck Contraction

POSITION A: With your head tilted back and hands placed on your forehead as shown, begin pushing up and forward against the resistance of your hands. Maintain peak contraction for 7 to 12 seconds while following correct breathing procedure. Relax.

POSITIONS B AND C: Repeat exercise as described above. Relax. Take 7 to 10 power breaths and move to exercise #3.

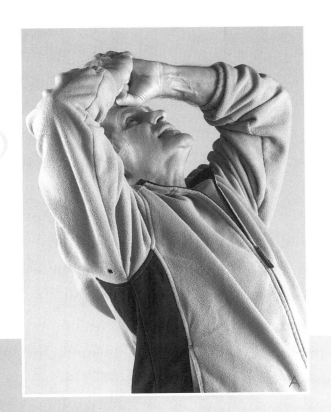

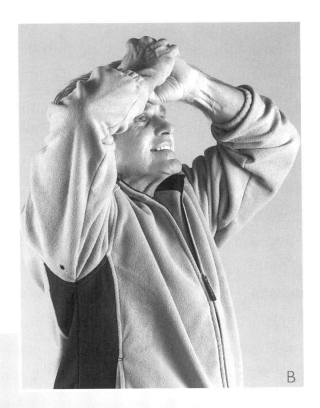

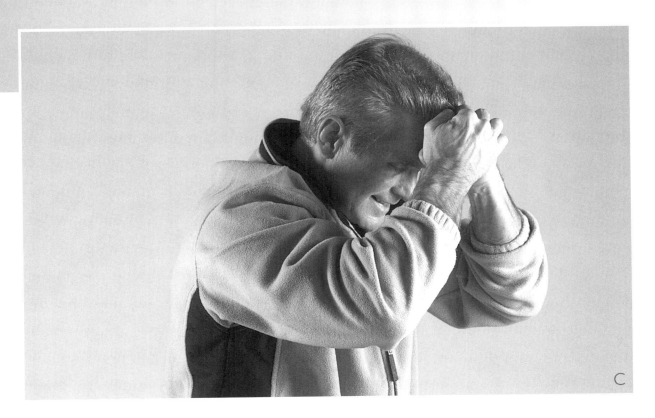

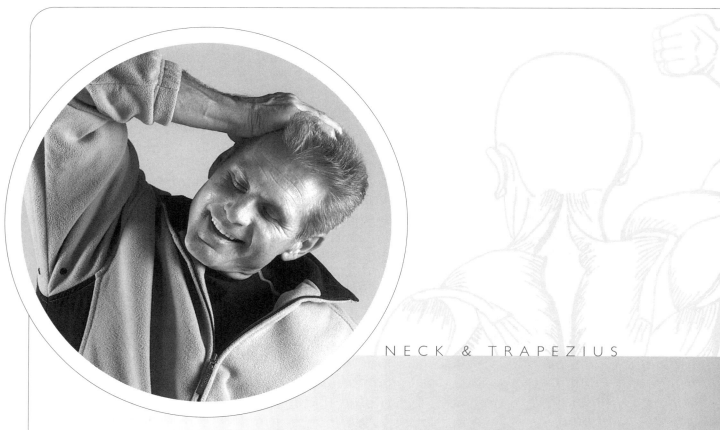

NECK EXERCISE #3
Side Neck Contraction (left to right)

POSITION A: With the left side of your head close to your left shoulder, place your right hand on the right side of your head as shown. Begin pushing your head to the right side while resisting with your right hand. Maintain intensity for 7 to 12 seconds while following the correct breathing procedure. Relax. Breathe deeply and then repeat in positions B and C.

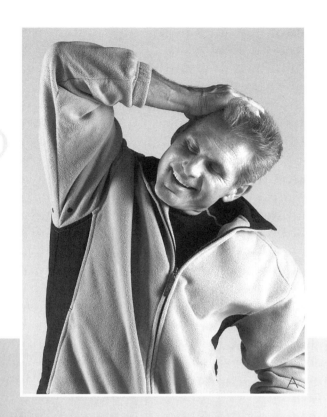

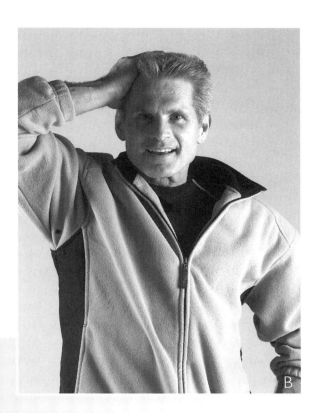

POSITIONS

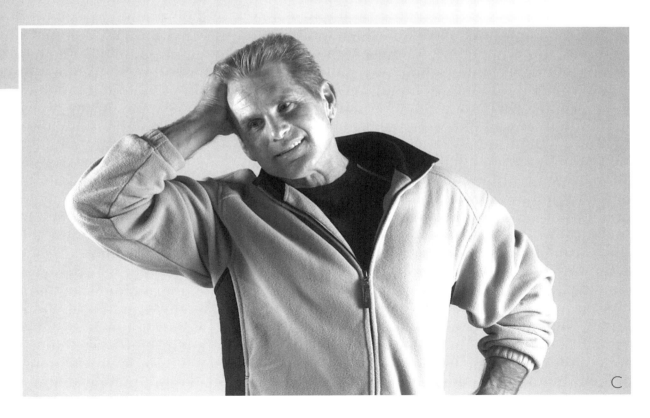

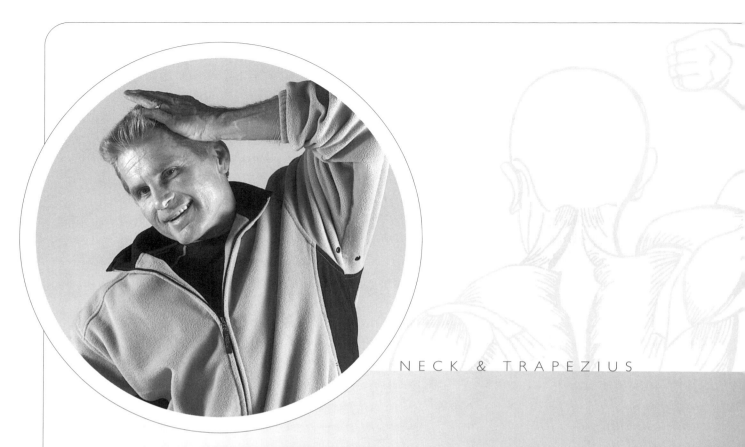

NECK EXERCISE #4
Side Neck Contraction *(right to left)*

POSITION A, B, AND C: Follow the exact same procedures as in Neck Exercise #3, moving from right to left while following the correct breathing procedure in all three positions. Relax. Take 10 power breaths and proceed to exercise #5.

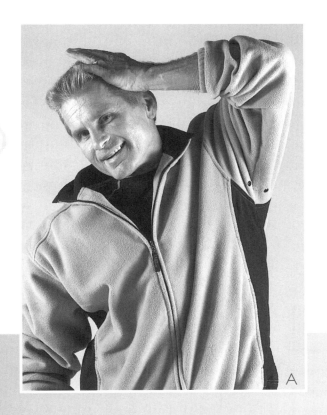

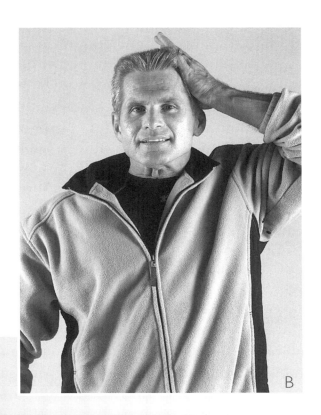

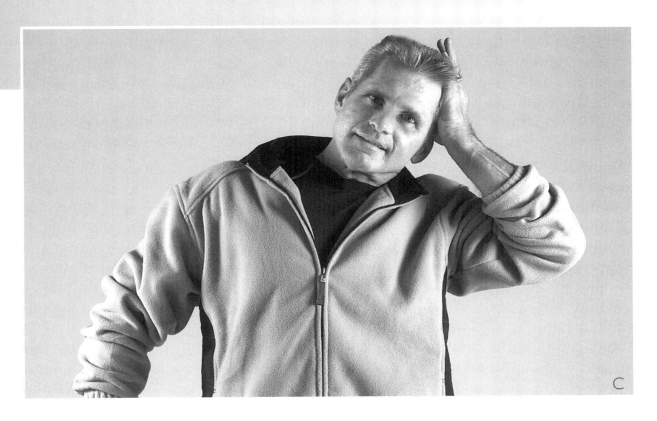

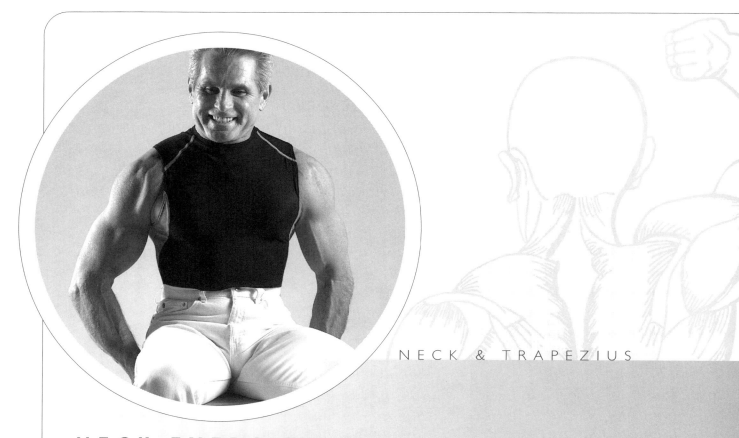

NECK EXERCISE #5
Trapezius Contraction

In the previous 4 exercises, we have exercised the neck and trapezius muscles together. In this final exercise for this series, we will isolate the trapezius for one intense contraction.

Sit in a chair with your feet approximately 12" apart. Grasp the bottom of the chair seat with your hands (as shown) and bring your shoulders upward until your arms are fully extended. Follow the correct breathing procedure while working to achieve the maximum contraction. Then slowly begin exhaling while making an *f-f-f-f* or *s-s-s-s* sound, maintaining your peak contraction for 7 to 12 seconds. Slowly release your contraction for 3 to 4 seconds while breathing in. Relax.

Congratulations! You have just completed the entire neck and trapezius series.

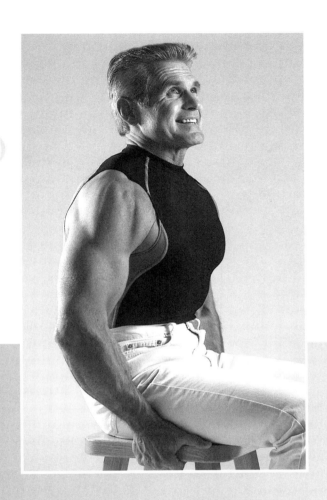
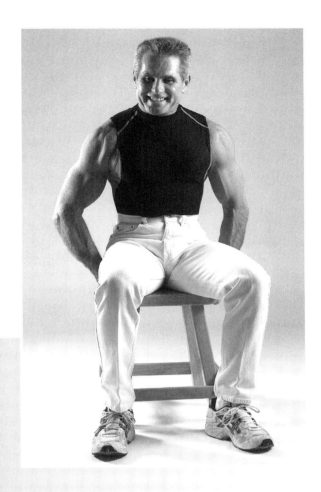

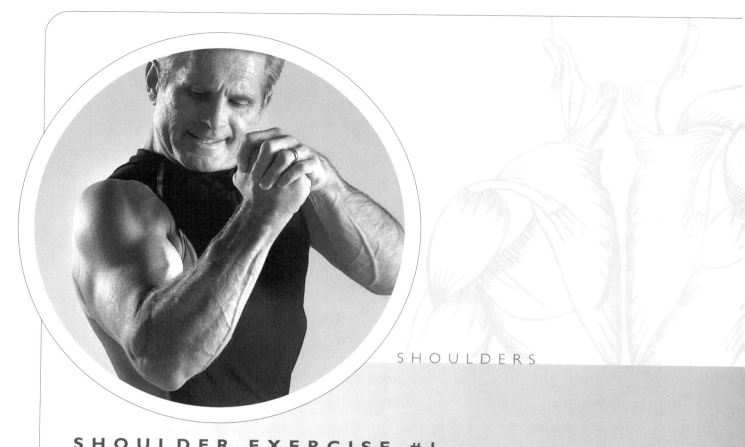

SHOULDER EXERCISE #1
One Arm Press

POSITION A: Stand erect with your feet about 12" apart. Clench your right fist as tightly as possible and bend your elbow as shown so that your right fist is in front of your right shoulder. Place your left hand over your right fist. Now slowly begin pushing upward with your right fist while resisting with your left hand. Build to peak intensity for 3 to 4 seconds, maintain maximum tension for 7 to 12 seconds, and then slowly release while following the proper breathing procedure.

After 7 to 10 power breaths, repeat the exercise from the *left side*, following the exact same procedure as outlined above.

POSITION B: Repeat the exercise as described above, but raise your right fist to forehead level. Once again, build and maintain your contraction while following the correct breathing procedure. Relax. Power breathe and switch to left side and repeat.

POSITION C: Repeat the exercise as shown in position C with arms near full extension. Switch sides and repeat, always following the correct breathing procedure.

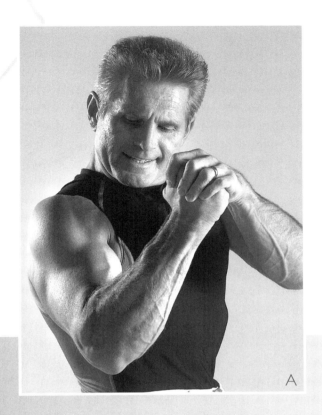

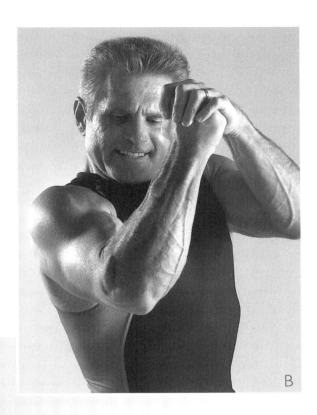

POSITIONS

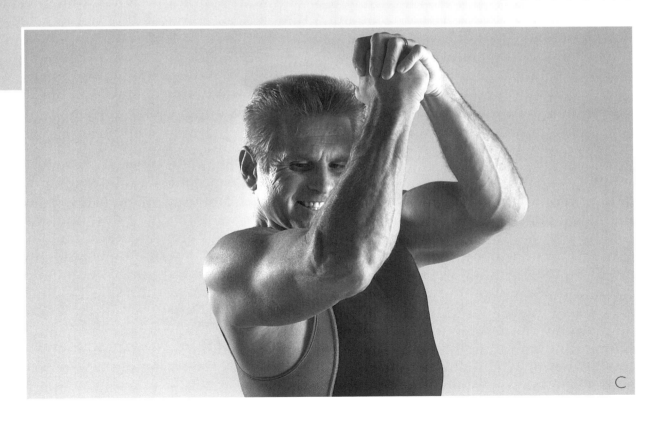

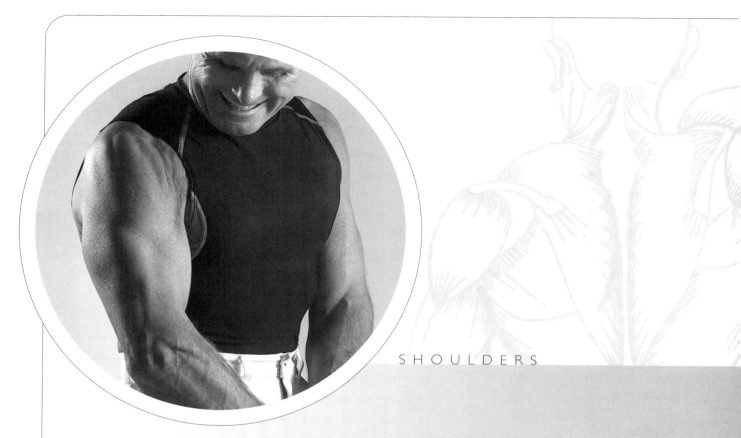

SHOULDERS

SHOULDER EXERCISE #2
Front Deltoid Contraction

POSITION A: Stand erect with your feet about 12" apart. Clench your right fist as powerfully as possible. Grasp the back of your right wrist with your left hand about 6" in front of your right thigh. Keeping your arm straight, push your right hand firmly upward while powerfully resisting with your left hand. Slowly build the tension while following correct breathing procedures. Maintain maximum tension for 7 to 12 seconds. Relax. Power breathe, then switch sides and repeat.

POSITION B: Repeat the exercise as described above, and elevate your right arm to just above waist level. Upon completion, switch hands to right over left and repeat.

POSITION C: Follow the same procedures as outlined above, only your right fist is about shoulder level or just slightly below. Once again, maintain the maximum tension for 7 to 12 seconds, then switch hands with your right over left and repeat the entire procedure with focused breathing as outlined previously. Relax. Practice power breathing, then move on to exercise #3.

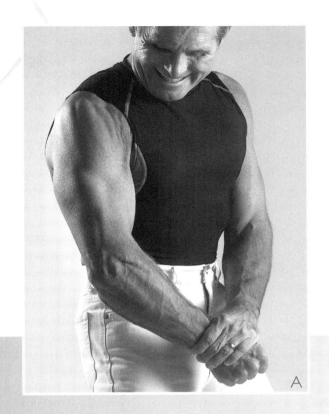

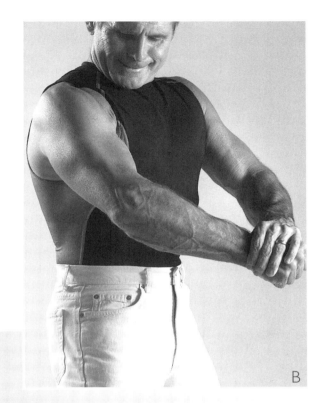

POSITIONS

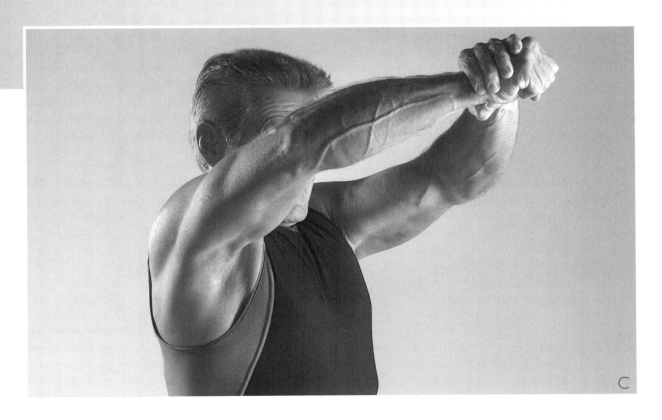

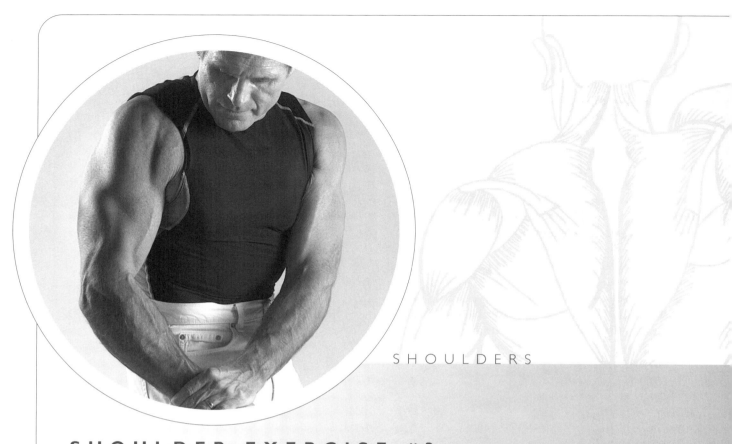

SHOULDER EXERCISE #3
Side Deltoid Raise

POSITION A, B, AND C: Observe the photos showing each position. Note that we are raising our arm diagonally out to the side. Position A begins about 6" away from the right thigh; position B is at approximately waist level, and position C is at approximately shoulder level or slightly below. Follow the correct breathing protocols and hold your peak contraction for 7 to 12 seconds in each position. Remember to perform all three contractions from both sides of the body.

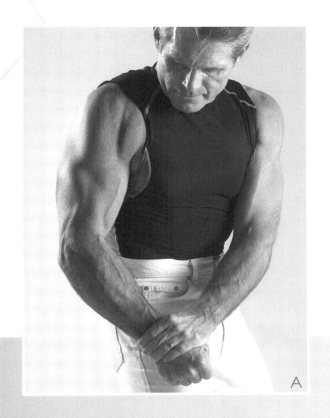

A

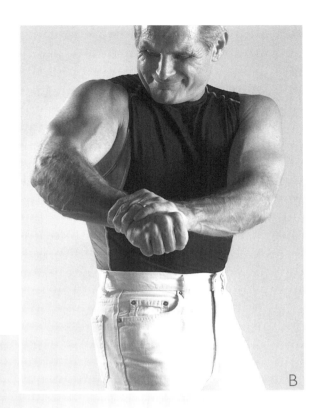

B

POSITIONS

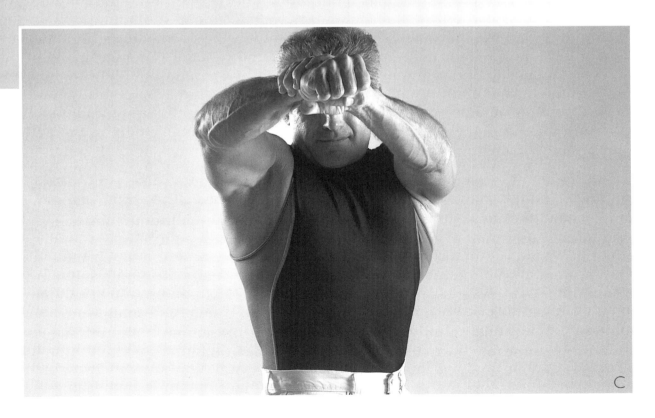

C

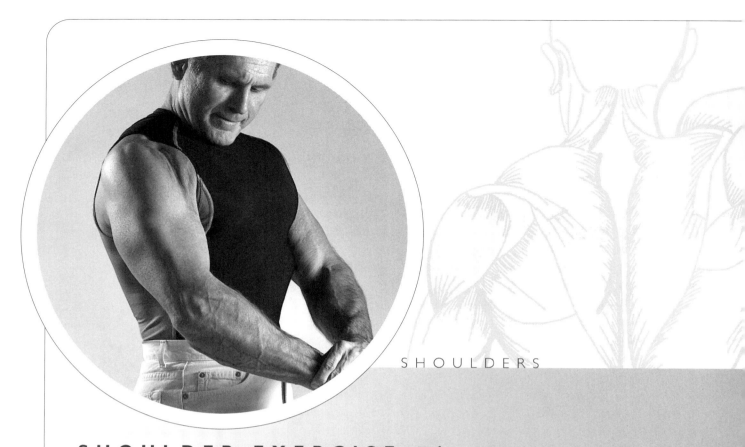

SHOULDER EXERCISE #4
Back Deltoid Contraction

POSITION A, B, AND C: Study the photos carefully. We start with the right hand 6" from the body and directly at the centerline, with your left hand grasping the back of your right hand. This time, however, we endeavor to pull the right arm directly sideways and back. As you will soon discover, you will feel an intense contraction in the rear deltoid muscle. Upon reaching maximum contraction, hold it for 7 to 12 seconds. Then switch hands with your right hand over your left hand and repeat, endeavoring to pull your left arm directly to the left side and back.

Be sure to follow the correct breathing procedure during all CICs. That means to slowly build tension while deeply inhaling for 3 to 4 seconds, holding the peak contraction for 7 to 12 seconds while exhaling slowly and making an *f-f-f-f* or *s-s-s-s* sound (it sounds like air being let out of a tire), and finally slowly releasing tension for 3 to 4 seconds while inhaling. Then relax. Power breathe for 7 to 10 breaths and continue to positions B and C and be sure to exercise both shoulders equally.

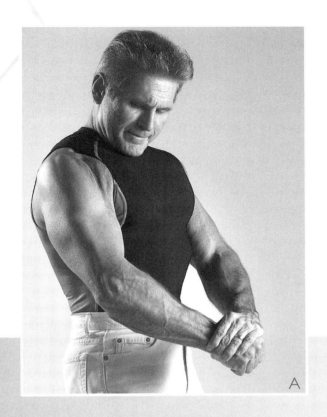

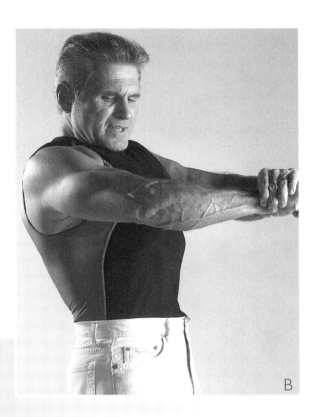

POSITIONS

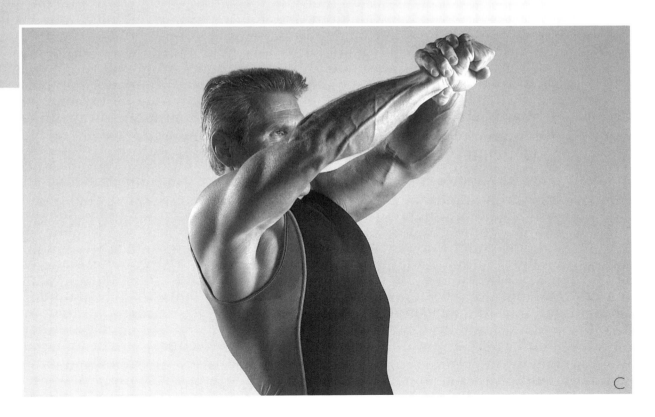

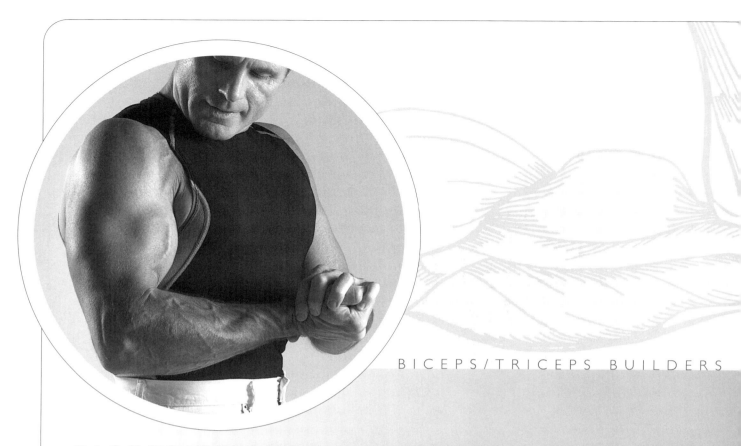

BICEPS/TRICEPS EXERCISE #1
Biceps Curl

POSITION A: Stand erect with your feet about 12" apart. With your right arm at the right side of your body and slightly bent at the right elbow, clench your right fist tightly. Place your left hand over your right fist as shown. Pull your right fist toward your right shoulder while powerfully resisting with your left hand. Slowly build tension for 3 to 4 seconds while inhaling. Hold your peak contraction 7 to 12 seconds while slowly exhaling and making an *f-f-f-f* or *s-s-s-s* sound. Then slowly release the contraction another 3 to 4 seconds while inhaling slowly. Relax. Power breathe. Then repeat with your left side following the exact same procedures outlined above.

POSITION B: Same exercise as above only the angle is changed so that your clenched fist is at about 90°. Follow the exact same protocols as in position A. Upon completion, repeat the contraction with your right hand over your left fist.

POSITION C: Repeat the exercise as described above. This time raise your right fist to a position parallel to your right shoulder with your arm bent at the elbow. Maintain peak intensity for 7 to 12 seconds while following the correct breathing protocols. Relax and repeat with your left arm.

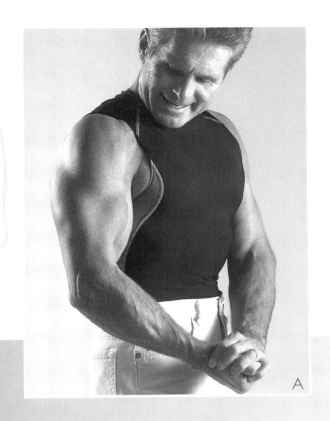

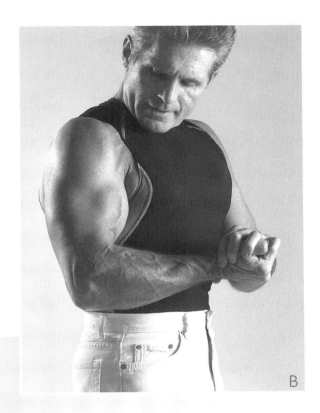

POSITIONS

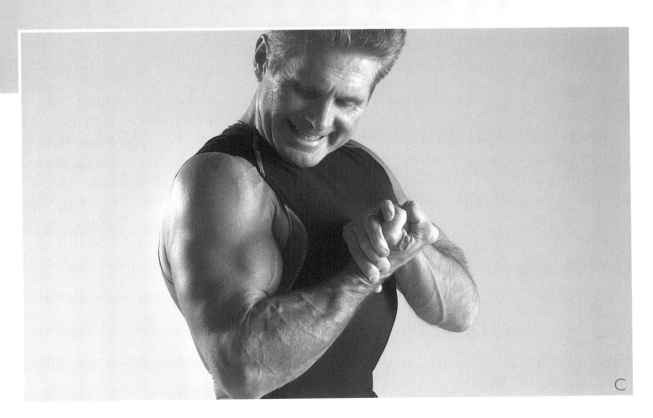

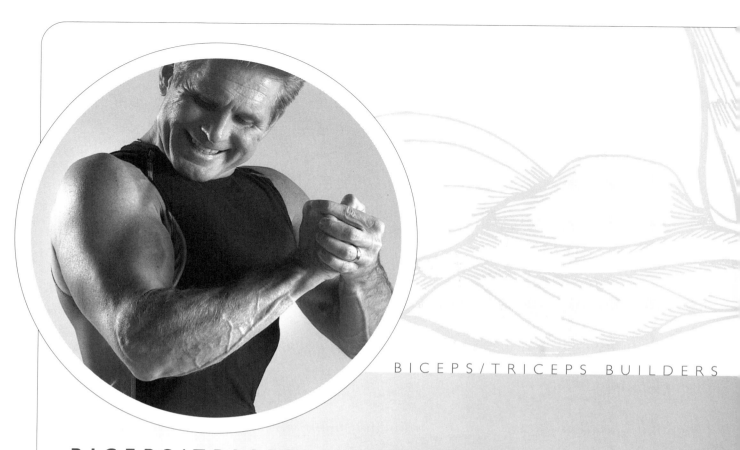

BICEPS/TRICEPS EXERCISE #2
Triceps Press Down

POSITION A: Stand erect with your feet about 12" apart. With your elbow bent, clench your right fist (fingers facing down) and hold your fist in front of your right shoulder. Grasp your right fist with your left hand as shown. Press downward powerfully while resisting with your left hand. Slowly build tension for 3 to 4 seconds while inhaling. Hold your peak intensity for 7 to 12 seconds while slowly exhaling and making an *f-f-f-f* or *s-s-s-s* sound. Then slowly release the contraction for another 3 to 4 seconds while inhaling slowly. Relax. Perform 7 to 10 power breaths. Then repeat with your left fist while resisting with your right hand.

POSITION B: Repeat the exercise exactly as described above, but lower the right fist to about a 90° angle as shown in the photo. Follow the exact same protocols for breathing, contracting, and releasing the contraction. Upon completion, repeat the contraction with your right hand resisting your left fist.

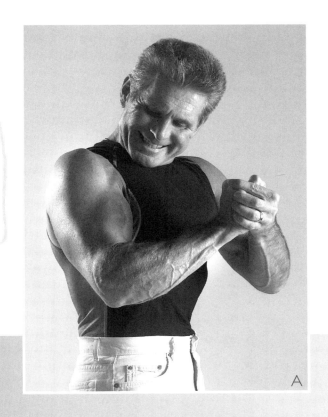

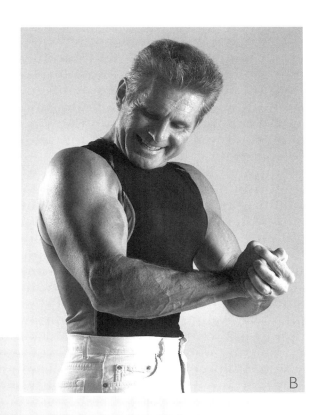

POSITION C: Follow the exact same protocols as given in positions A and B. This time, however, begin with your right fist approximately 7" lower than in position B. Grasp your right fist as shown and powerfully press down while resisting mightily with your left hand. Follow the same breathing, contracting, and releasing protocols. Relax. Perform 7 to 10 power breaths. Then finish up by repeating position C with your left fist while resisting with your right hand.

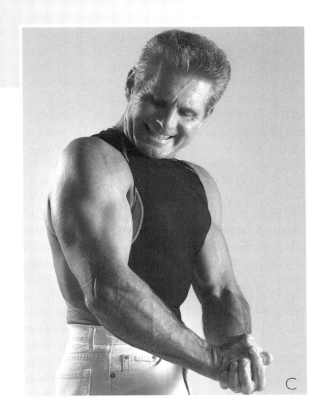

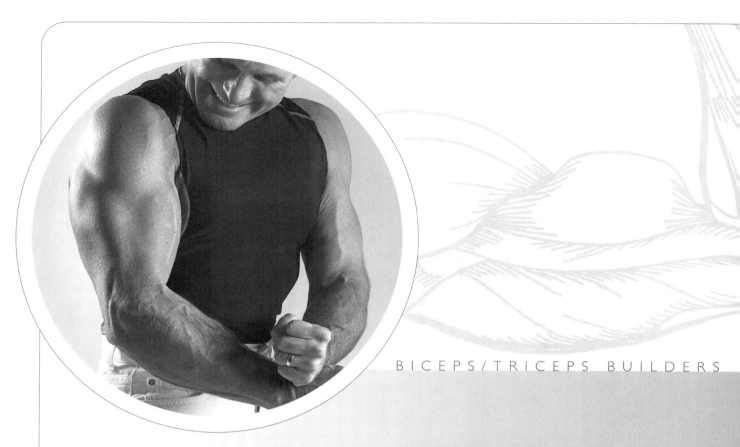

BICEPS/TRICEPS EXERCISE #3
"The Milo" Biceps/Triceps Contraction

You may remember what I wrote previously about my uncle Milo having the most perfectly developed physique I've ever seen. He was 6'3", 210 pounds, and literally looked like what you'd expect the Super Hero "Doc Savage" to look like. Just as the Doc Savage books clearly stated that Doc developed his incredible strength and physique by following Charles Atlas's Dynamic Tension Methods, so did my uncle Milo. And though I've seen many men over the years who had bigger and bulkier arms than my uncle, not one has ever come close to the perfectly sculpted look of my uncle's arms. After he started performing the Atlas exercises in an Isometric fashion, he came up with this biceps/triceps contraction that I have never seen anywhere else. For many men and women, it quickly becomes their favorite arm-developing exercise because it fully engages every muscle group of the entire hand-and-arm structure. In addition, because the muscles are worked directly in the centerline of the body, many people discover they can apply maximum levels of contraction more easily because of greatly enhanced leverage.

Here's how "The Milo" is done.

POSITION A: Stand erect with your feet about 12" apart. Clench both fists as tightly as possible and place them as shown with your left fist over your right at close to full extension

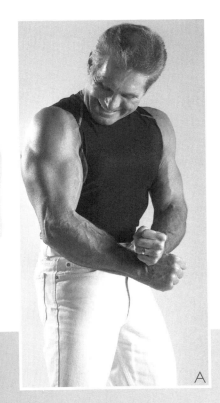
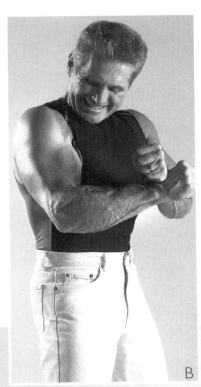
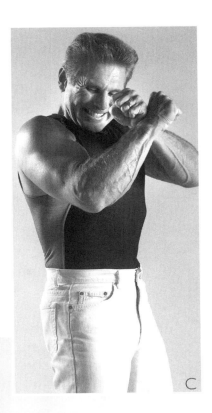

about 6" from the centerline of the body. With your right arm pulling up and your left arm pressing down, slowly build tension in both arms while inhaling for 3 to 4 seconds until you reach maximum contraction. Hold this maximum contraction for 7 to 12 seconds, slowly exhaling and making an *f-f-f-f* or *s-s-s-s* sound. Then slowly release the tension for another 3 to 4 seconds while inhaling slowly. Relax. Power breathe, then switch arms to right over left, following the exact same breathing and contraction procedures outlined above.

POSITION B: Follow the exact procedures as outlined in position A, with your left fist over your right, but this time begin the contraction with your arms at about 90°. Utilize the same breathing and contraction protocols as stated previously on this and all CIC exercises. Upon completion, switch the positions of your fists and continue with your right fist over the left.

POSITION C: Repeat the above exercise with your arms in position as shown. Your left fist is over the right and directly in front of the sternum in the centerline of the body. Your left fist will be about 6" from your body. Follow the correct breathing and contraction procedures outlined above. Upon completion, relax. Power breathe, and then continue with one final contraction starting with your right fist over the left.

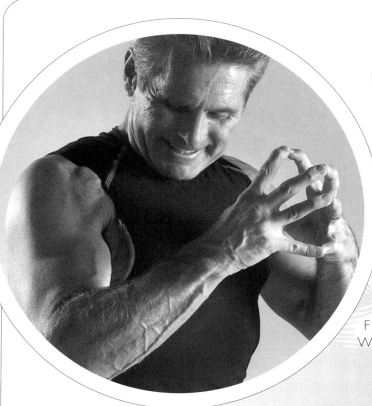

A Must for All Athletes and Sportsmen

FOR SUPER STRONG FINGERS,
WRISTS, AND FOREARMS

FINGERS, WRISTS, AND FOREARMS
Exercise #1

POSITION A, B, AND C: Stand erect with your feet about 12" apart. Bring the tips of the fingers on both of your hands together, about 3" away from the center of your chest. Spread your fingers wide and press the fingertips of your right hand and left hands firmly together. Slowly inhale for 3 to 4 seconds while increasing the tension in the opposing fingers to the maximum. Hold the contraction for 7 to 12 seconds while slowly exhaling and making an *f-f-f-f* or *s-s-s-s* sound. Slowly inhale for another 3 to 4 seconds while releasing tension. Relax. Power breathe, then move on to exercise #2.

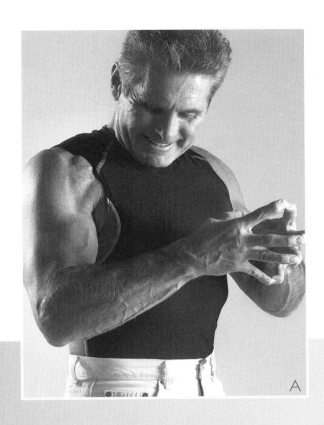

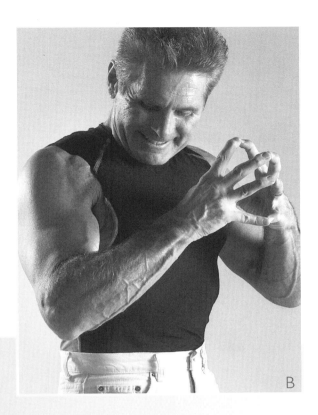

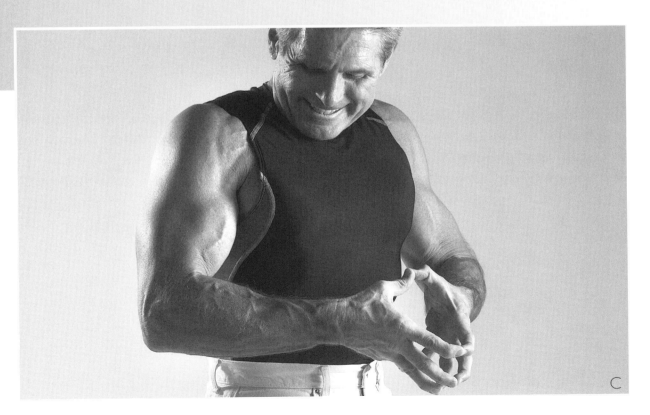

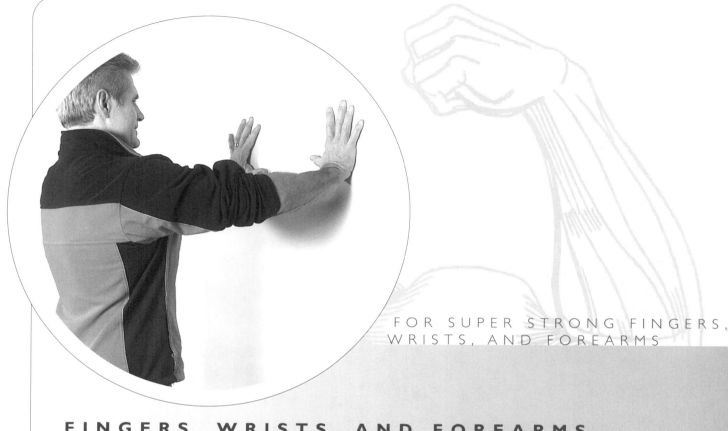

FINGERS, WRISTS, AND FOREARMS
Exercise #2

POSITION A, B, AND C: Stand erect with your feet about 12" apart and approximately 3' from a wall. Place the fingertips of both hands against the wall with hands about 12" apart while keeping your arms straight. Press firmly against the wall while applying correct breathing and contraction procedures. Upon completion, relax. Power breathe and continue on to exercise #3.

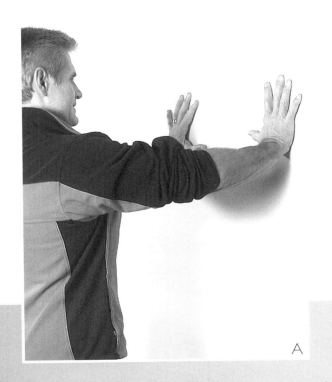

A

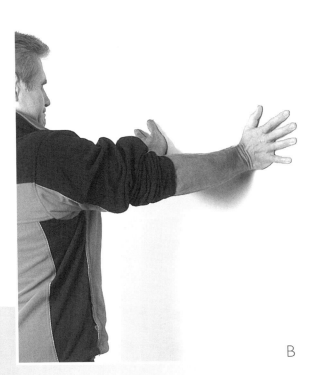

B

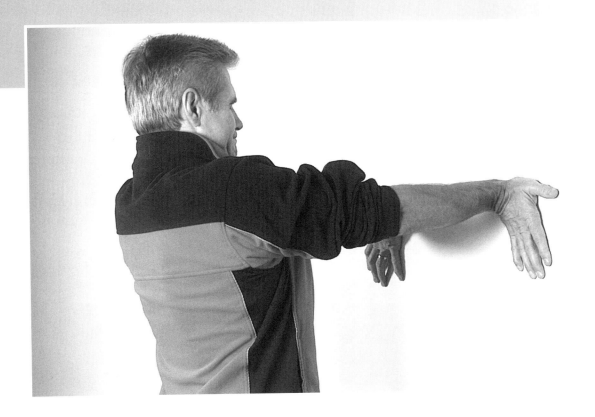

C

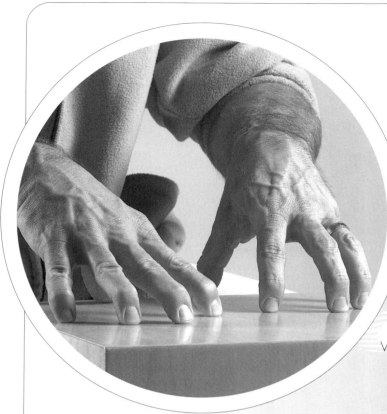

FINGERS, WRISTS, AND FOREARMS
Exercise #3

POSITION A, B, AND C: Sit in a chair facing a table or desk. Place the fingertips of both your hands on the edge of the table or desk. Press your fingertips firmly downward and build in intensity while inhaling for 3 to 4 seconds. Hold the peak intensity for 7 to 12 seconds, exhaling slowly while making an *f-f-f-f* or *s-s-s-s* sound. Slowly release pressure for 3 to 4 seconds while breathing in. Relax. Take 7 to 10 power breaths, then move on to exercise #4.

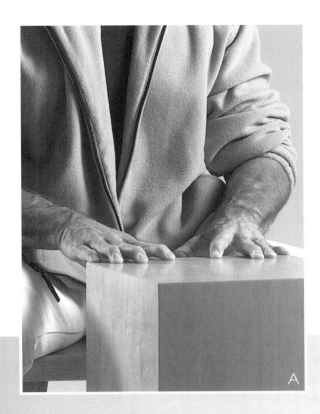

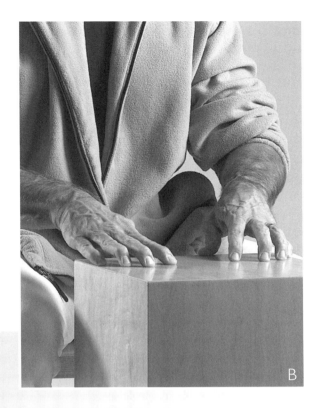

POSITIONS

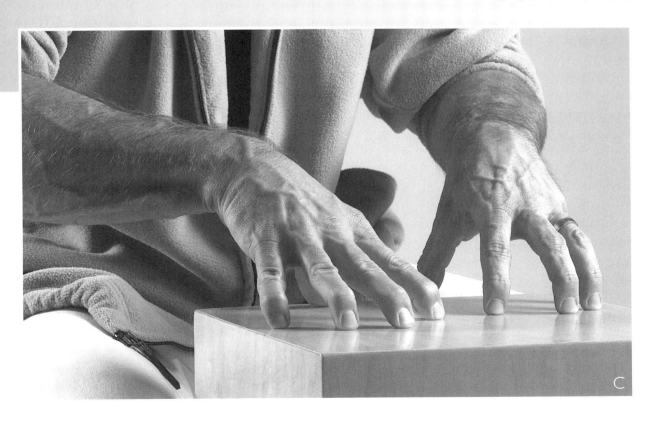

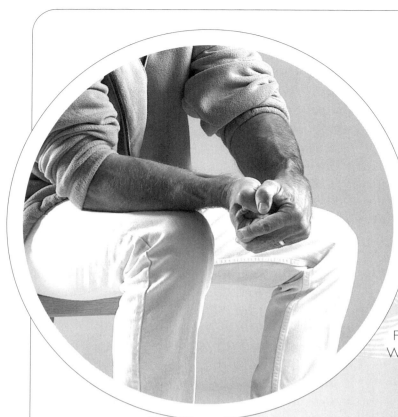

FINGERS, WRISTS, AND FOREARMS
Exercise #4

POSITION A, B, AND C: Sit in a chair. Place the back of your right forearm on your right thigh (palm facing up) with the hand extending over your right knee. Clench your right hand into a tight fist, powerfully flexing your wrist and contracting your right forearm muscles. Place your left hand over your right as shown. Pull your right fist upward while firmly resisting with your left hand. All the while, practice the correct breathing and contraction protocol as given in the previous exercises. Upon completion, relax. Power breathe 7 to 10 repetitions and then perform the same contraction with your left wrist and forearm, resisting with your right hand.

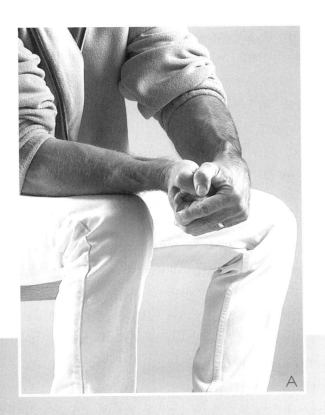

A

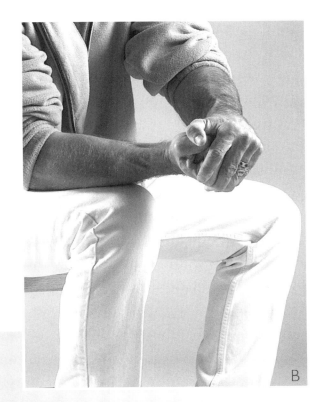

B

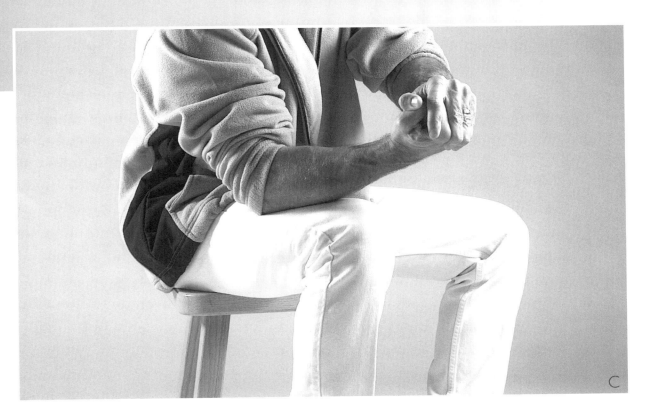

C

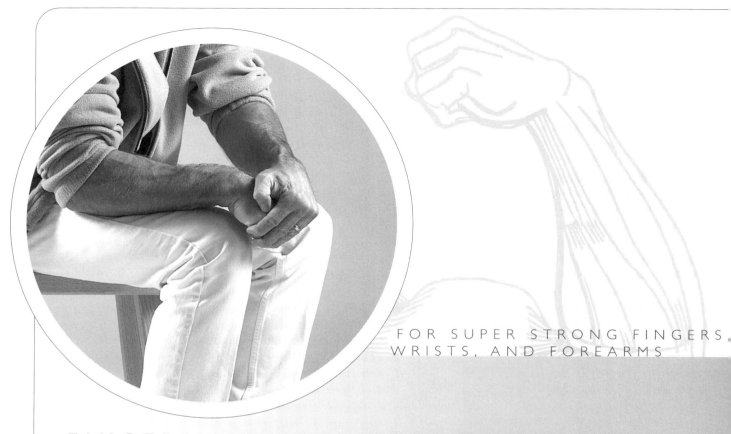

FOR SUPER STRONG FINGERS,
WRISTS, AND FOREARMS

FINGERS, WRISTS, AND FOREARMS
Exercise #5

POSITION A, B, AND C: Repeat exercise #4, but this time the underside of your forearm will be in contact with your right thigh, and your palm will be facing down. Place your left hand over your right (the back of this fist this time) and endeavor to flex your wrist back and up while following the correct breathing and contraction protocols given previously. Take 10 to 12 power breaths and repeat with your right hand resisting the left fist. When finished, take 10 power breaths and finish up with exercise #6.

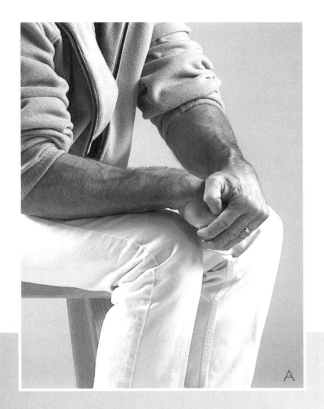

A

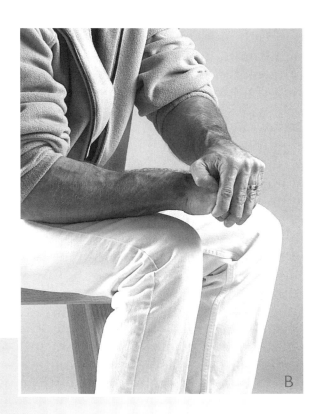

B

POSITIONS

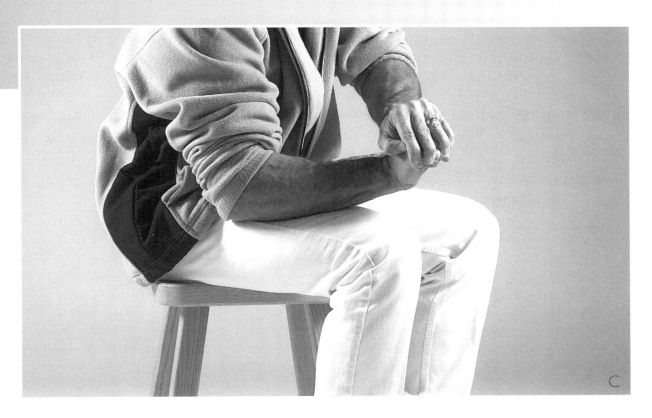

C

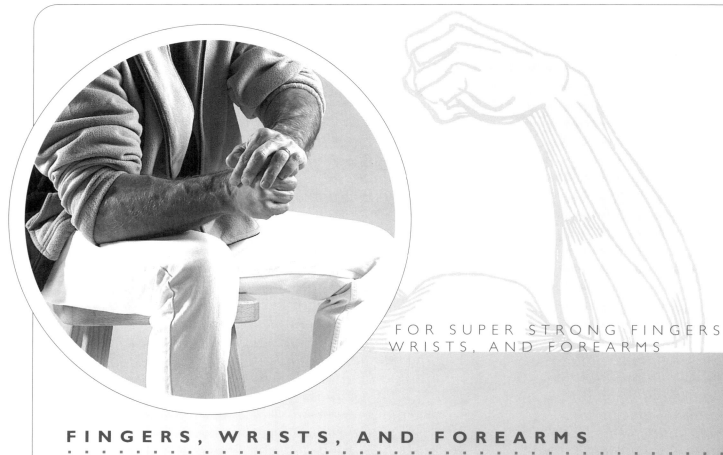

FINGERS, WRISTS, AND FOREARMS
Exercise #6

POSITION A, B, AND C: Repeat exercises #4 and 5, but this time your fist and forearm will be sideways with your thumb and forefinger facing up. While supplying powerful resistance from your left hand, endeavor to flex your right fist up. Practice the correct breathing and contraction protocols. Relax. Power breathe and then perform the same exercises on your left side. When completed, practice 7 to 10 more power breaths before continuing.

Now that we have worked the muscles of our neck, trapezius, shoulders, upper arms, wrists, fingers, and forearms, we are ready to focus directly upon the pectoral muscles of the chest.

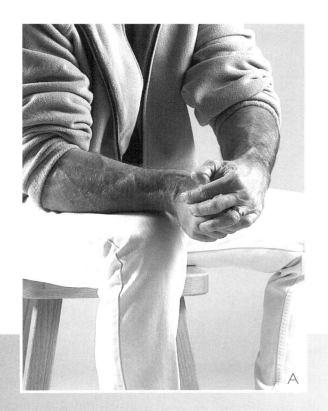

A

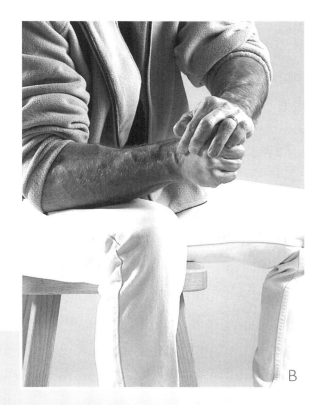

B

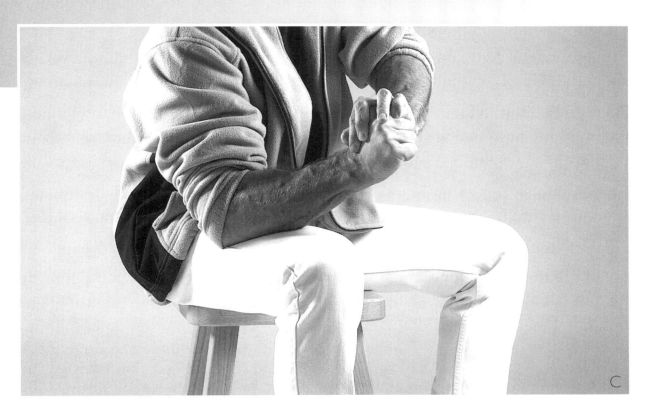

C

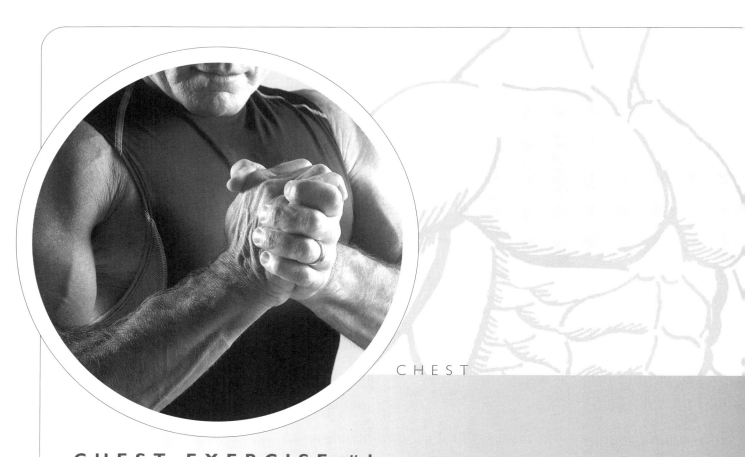

CHEST

CHEST EXERCISE #1
Pectoral Contraction for the Mid Chest

POSITIONS A, B, AND C: Stand erect with your feet about 12" apart. Clasp your hands at the center of your chest as shown with the fingers of your right hand in the top position between the thumb and forefinger of your left hand. Extend your elbows outward and slightly away from your chest. Press your hands firmly against each other while slowly building tension as you inhale for 3 to 4 seconds until you reach maximum contraction. At that point, slowly begin a controlled exhale for 7 to 12 seconds while maintaining a maximum muscular contraction. Then slowly release the tension as you inhale deeply for 3 to 4 seconds. Relax. Take 7 to 10 deep power breaths, and then repeat the exercise while changing the relative positions of your hands with the fingers of your left hand in the top position between the thumb and forefinger of your right hand. Follow the breathing and contraction procedures outlined above. Relax. Take 10 power breaths and move to exercise #2.

NOTE: On all the chest contractions you can also perform two additional contractions by placing your left fist in the palm of your right hand and completing the contraction. Then reverse it with your right fist in your left palm. Obviously, all 4 pectoral contractions build your arms, back, and abs as well as other supportive muscular structures.

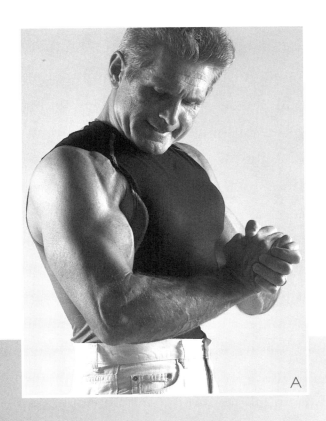

A

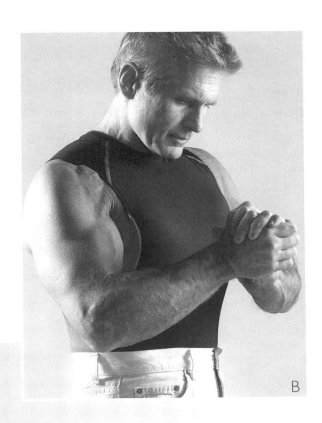

B

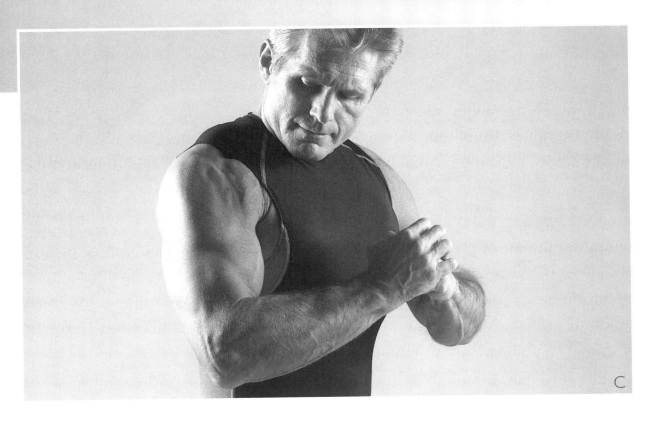

C

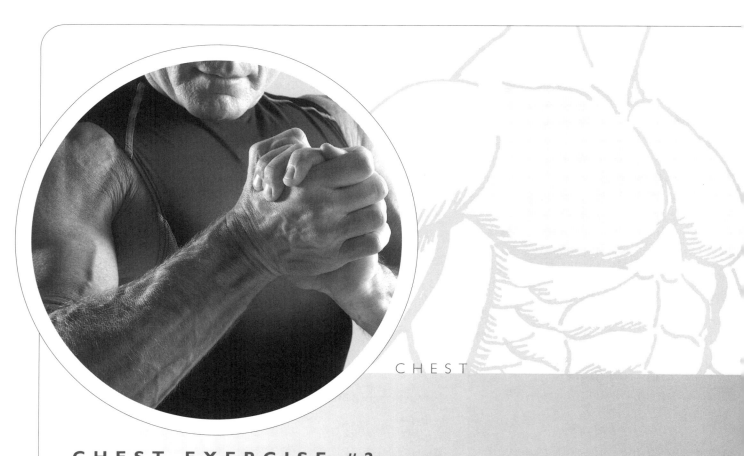

CHEST

CHEST EXERCISE #2
Pectoral Contraction #2

POSITIONS A, B, AND C: Same exercise in concept as exercise #1 except this time we raise our arms to just below chin level in front of the center of our neck. Clasp your hands so that the right hand occupies the top position with the fingers of your right hand between the thumb and forefingers of your left hand.

Perform the exercise exactly as described previously. Upon completion, relax. Power breathe, then repeat with your left hand occupying the top position with the fingers of your left hand between the thumb and forefingers of your right hand. Remember to follow the exact breathing and contraction protocols for this and all other CIC exercises. That means:

- 3 to 4 seconds inhalation while building to maximum contraction.
- 7 to 12 seconds maintaining a maximum contraction while exhaling slowly and making an *f-f-f-f* or *s-s-s-s* sound.
- Inhale slowly for another 3 to 4 seconds while releasing the tension.
- Relax. Take 7 to 10 power breaths.

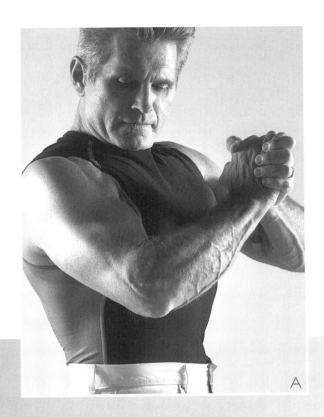

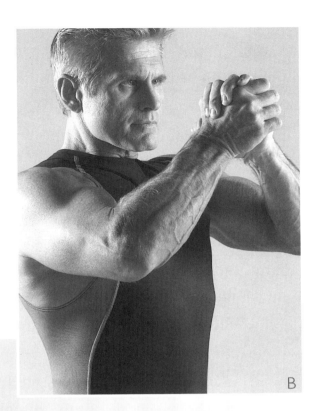

POSITIONS

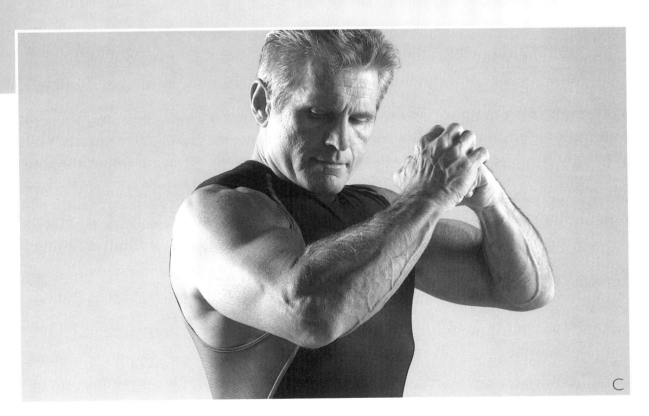

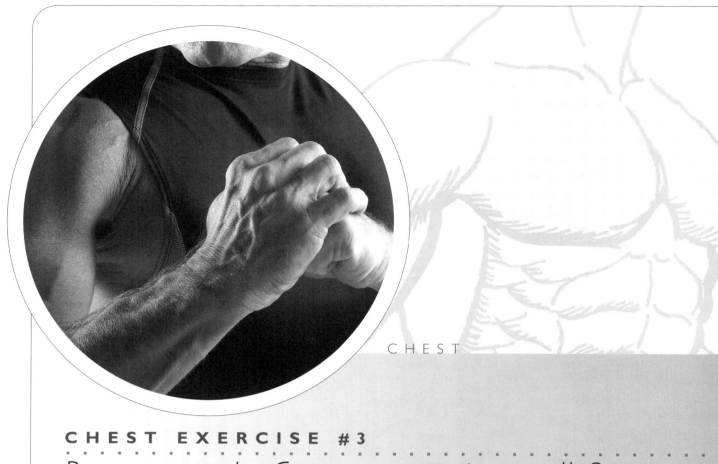

CHEST

CHEST EXERCISE #3
Pectoral Contraction #3

POSITIONS A, B, AND C: Study the photos. Note that this contraction begins at forehead level. Clasp your hands so that the right hand occupies the top position with the fingers of your right hand between the thumb and forefingers of your left hand. Follow the correct breathing and contraction protocols while intensifying the contractions for 3 to 4 seconds. Maintain a peak contraction for 7 to 12 seconds, practicing a controlled exhalation while making an *f-f-f-f* or *s-s-s-s* sound. And, finally, slowly inhale while releasing the tension for 3 to 4 seconds. Power breathe for 10 repetitions. Then repeat with your left hand occupying the top position with the fingers of your left hand between the thumb and forefingers of your right hand.

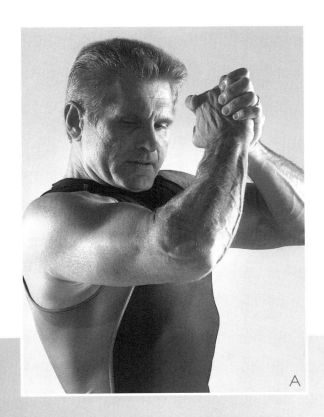

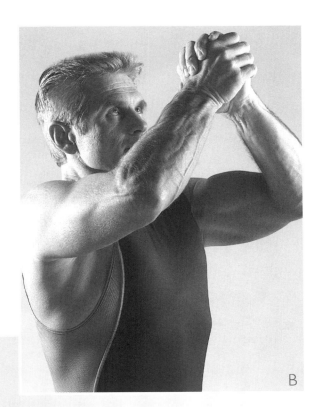

POSITIONS

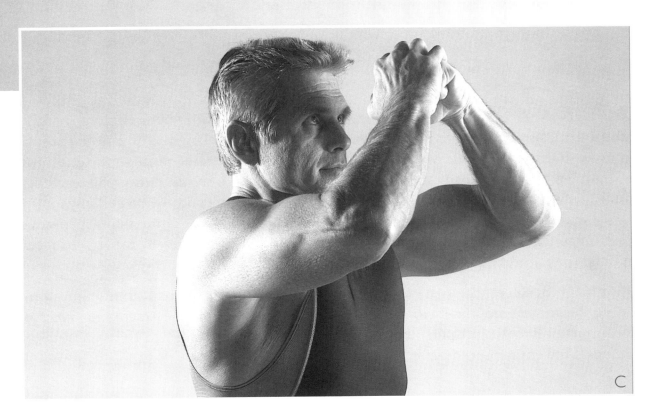

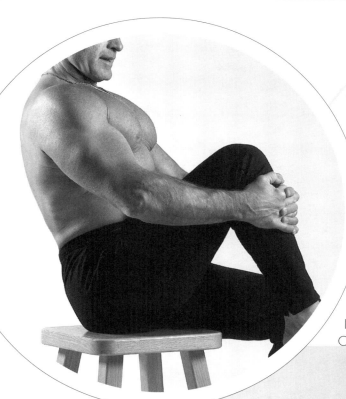

For a Wide "V" Shaped Back

LATISSIMUS DORSI MUSCLES
OF THE UPPER BACK

LATISSIMUS DORSI MUSCLES
Exercise #1

POSITION A: Sit erect on a chair. Bring your right knee up, with your right foot about 12" off the floor. Clasp both hands around your right knee, interlocking the fingers and keeping your arms straight. Now endeavor to pull your right knee back while resisting the effort with your right leg. Slowly intensify the effort while inhaling 3 to 4 seconds until you reach peak contraction. Begin a slowly controlled exhalation for 7 to 12 seconds while making an *f-f-f-f* or *s-s-s-s* sound and maintaining the intensity of the contraction the entire time. Then slowly release the tension as you inhale for 3 to 4 seconds. Relax. Power breathe for 7 to 10 repetitions, and then repeat the entire procedure on the left side.

POSITION B: Repeat the previous exercise but raise your right knee 4" to 6" higher while bending the arms appropriately for maximum contraction. Follow the exact same breathing and contraction protocols. Upon completion, relax. Power breathe for 7 to 10 repetitions, and then repeat the entire procedure on the left side.

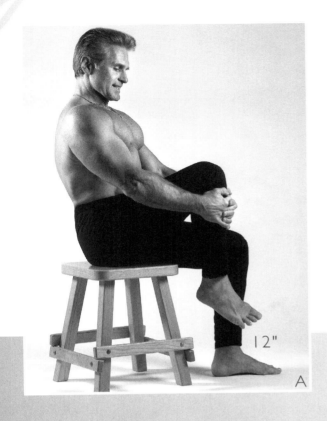

12" A

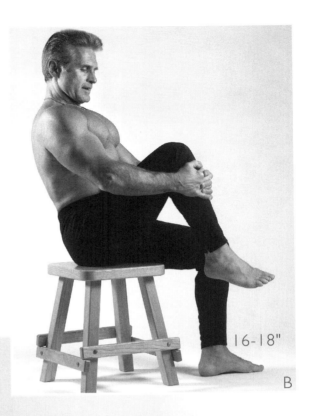

16-18" B

POSITION C: Repeat the exercise described above with the knee raised higher and the arms bent farther. Follow the same protocols for breathing and contraction. Upon completion, relax. Power breathe for 7 to 10 repetitions, and then perform one last repetition for the left side of the body.

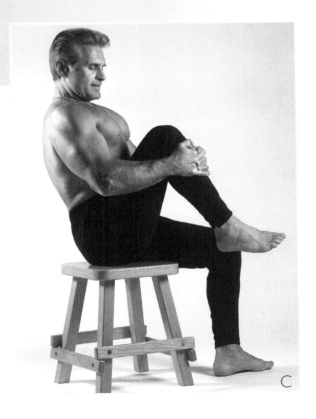

C

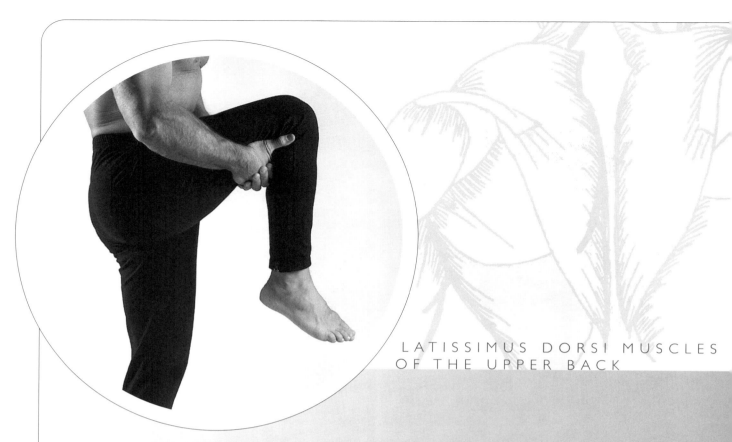

LATISSIMUS DORSI MUSCLES
Exercise #2

POSITION A: Bend forward from the waist as shown. Interlock the fingers of both your hands just above the backside of your right knee. With your arms pulling as shown, try to straighten your upper body against the resistance of your right leg. Slowly build tension while inhaling 3 to 4 seconds. Upon reaching peak contraction, begin a slowly controlled exhalation for 7 to 12 seconds while making an *f-f-f-f* or *s-s-s-s* sound and maintaining the intensity of the contraction the entire time. Then slowly release the tension while breathing in for another 3 to 4 seconds. Relax. Power breathe, and then repeat the entire procedure on the left side.

POSITION B: Repeat the previous exercise but raise your right knee and foot approximately 6" to 8" from the floor. Follow the correct breathing and contraction protocols. Upon completion, relax. Power breathe for 7 to 10 repetitions, then repeat the entire exercise on the left side.

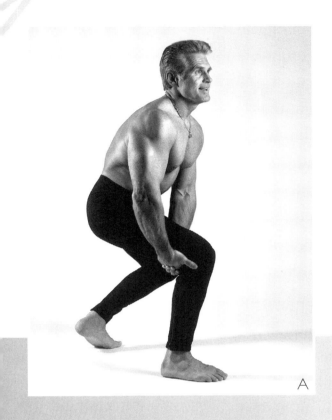

A

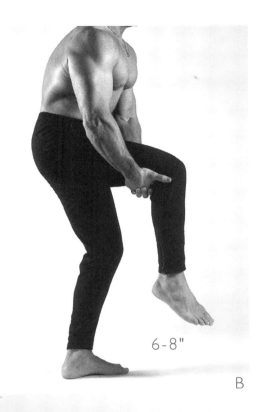

6-8"

B

POSITION C: Repeat the exercise described above except that your right knee is bent still farther and your right foot is now raised 12" to 16" from the floor. Follow the same protocols for breathing and contraction. Upon completion, relax. Power breathe, and then perform one last contraction on the left side of the body.

Pay special attention to this exercise because it also enhances balance in a big way.

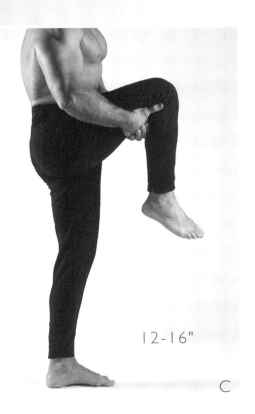

12-16"

C

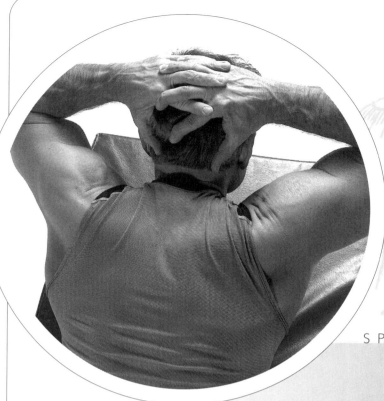

The following exercises for the erector spinal muscles yield exceptional results quickly and safely. This area is important to keep strong because the back ties into the abdominal area. Strong abs alone will not guarantee a pain-free back. But with these exercises, you'll go a long way toward remaining pain free for life.

SPINE

ERECTOR SPINAL MUSCLES
Exercise #1

Lie facedown on a mat, carpet, or bed with your feet close together, toes pointed, and head slightly raised. Place your hands behind your head, interlocking your fingers as shown. Now slowly inhale as you push upward firmly with both your head and shoulders for 3 to 4 seconds while resisting powerfully with your hands at the same time. As you achieve a peak contraction, slowly begin a controlled exhale, making an *f-f-f-f* or *s-s-s-s* sound for 7 to 12 seconds while maintaining the intensity of the contraction the entire time. Upon completion, slowly release the tension while inhaling 3 to 4 more seconds. Relax. Power breathe for 7 to 10 repetitions.

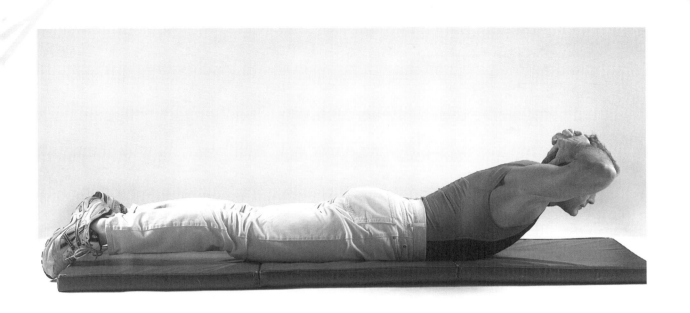

CORRECT HAND PLACEMENT

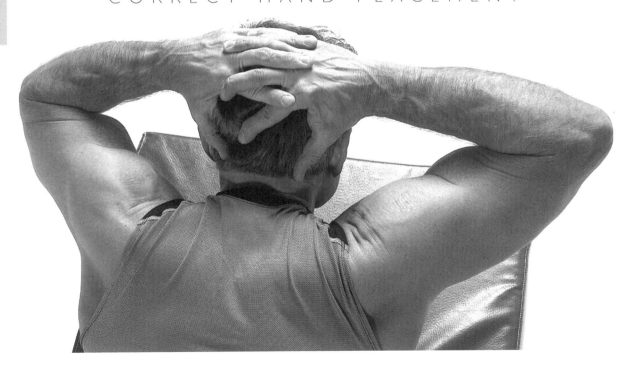

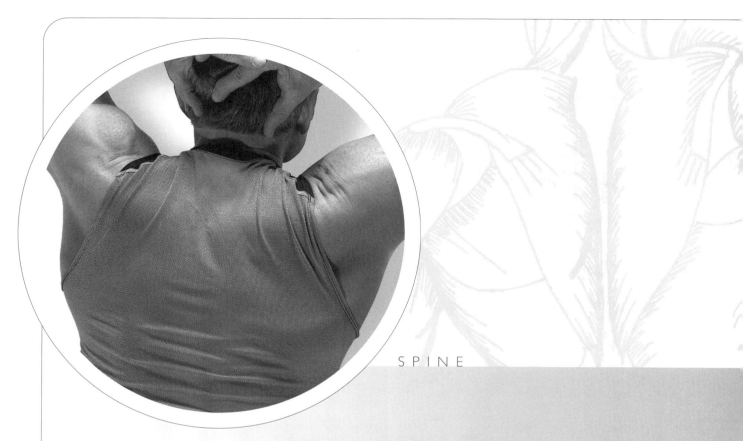

ERECTOR SPINAL MUSCLES
Exercise #2

While lying facedown on a stool or chair that is cushioned, place your hands behind your head and slowly raise both your head and feet upward while inhaling for 3 to 4 seconds and feeling the muscles in your lower back powerfully contract. Upon reaching peak contraction, slowly exhale for 7 to 12 seconds while making an *f-f-f-f* or *s-s-s-s* sound and maintaining the intensity of the contraction the entire time. Slowly release the tension for another 3 to 4 more seconds while breathing in. Relax. Take 7 to 10 power breaths.

The range of motion with this exercise is very short but very powerful. You may also perform the exercise with your arms straight in front of you. (And, no, you don't have to be Superman to do this, although you may look like him if you keep exercising!)

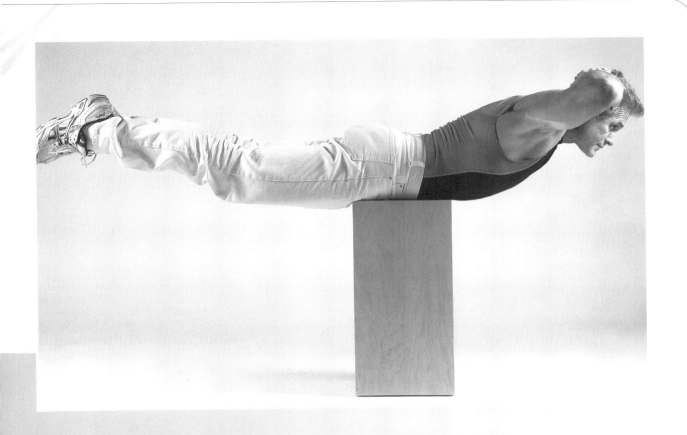

CORRECT HAND PLACEMENT

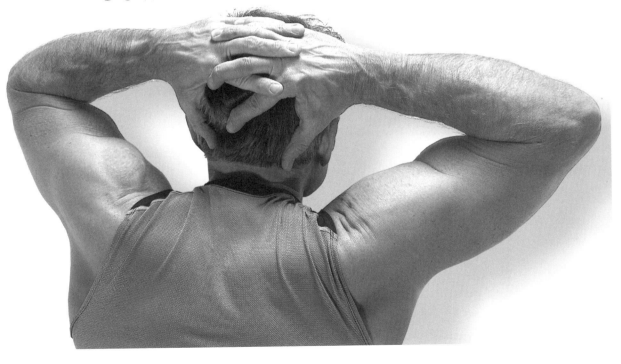

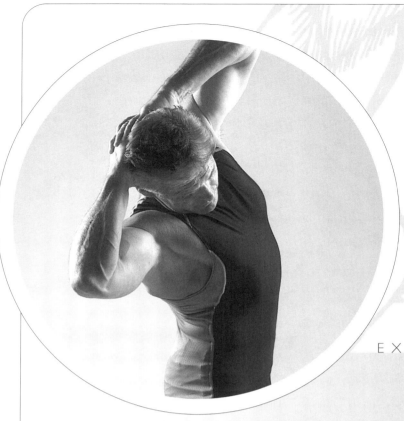

EXTERNAL OBLIQUES
Exercise #1

POSITION A: Stand erect with your feet about 12" apart. Place your hands behind your head and interlock your fingers. While inhaling slowly for 3 to 4 seconds, bend to the right until you feel the muscles in your right side powerfully contracting. At that point, slowly exhale for 7 to 12 seconds while maintaining peak contraction. Upon completion, slowly release the tension while inhaling for 3 to 4 seconds. Relax. Power breathe, then repeat on your left side.

POSITION B: Repeat the previous exercise following the exact same protocols except you'll start with your feet just 6" apart. (And, yes, this change of position makes a difference.) Be sure to complete on your left side as well.

POSITION C: Repeat the previous exercise except this time your feet will be together. Follow the same breathing and contraction protocols.

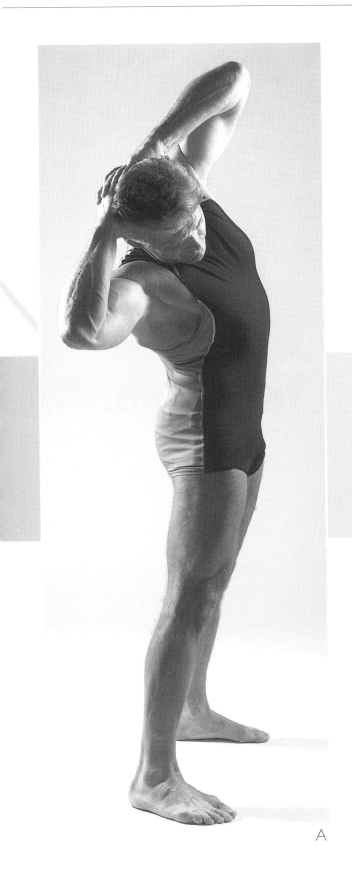

A

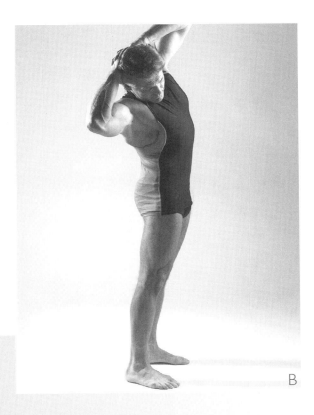

B

POSITIONS

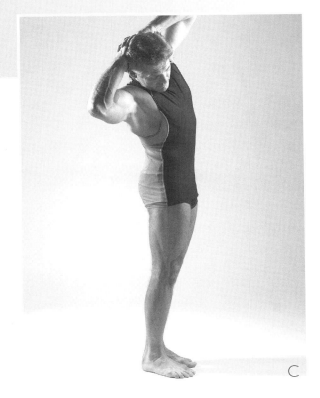

C

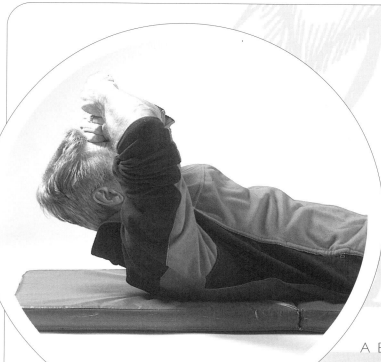

*To Strengthen and Firm
the Entire Abdominal Structure*

ABDOMINALS

ABDOMINALS EXERCISE #1
Iso Sit-Up

POSITION A, B, AND C: Lie on the floor with your feet together and toes pointed forward and down. Tightly clench your fists and position them on your forehead. Now raise your head and shoulders off the ground and endeavor to touch your chin to your chest as you inhale for 3 to 4 seconds while trying to sit up against the powerful resistance provided by your hands. You won't be able to sit up, but trying to do so will cause a powerful muscle contraction of the abdominal muscles. As you reach peak contraction of your rectus abdominis muscle, begin a slow controlled exhale for 7 to 12 seconds while maintaining as powerful a contraction as possible of your abdominal muscles. Upon completion, slowly release the tension for 3 to 4 seconds and relax completely.

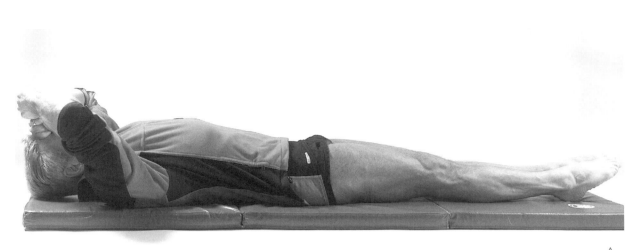

A

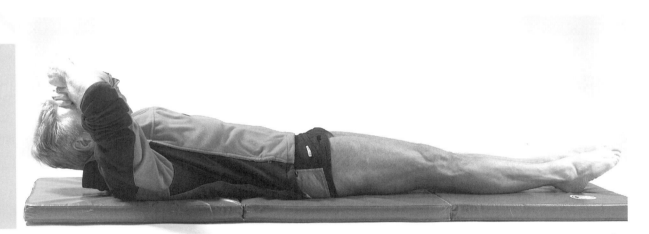

B

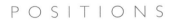

POSITIONS

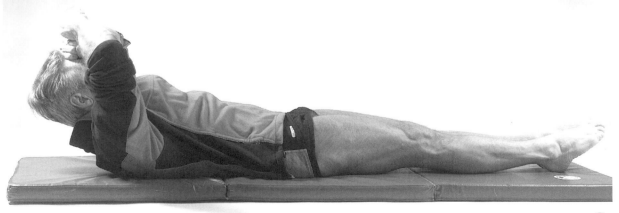

C

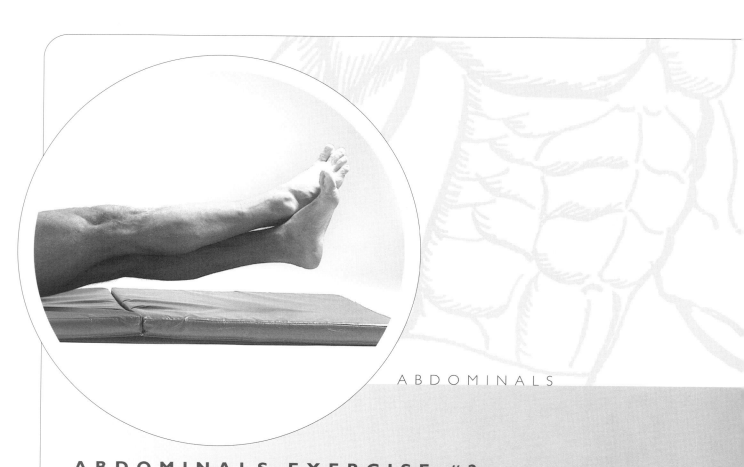

ABDOMINALS

ABDOMINALS EXERCISE #2
Iso Leg Raise for the Lower Abdominals

POSITION A, B, AND C: Lie on your back as in the previous exercise. Place your right foot over your left ankle. Raise both feet about 6" from the floor, bracing yourself as shown. While inhaling for 3 to 4 seconds, slowly press your left foot upward while powerfully resisting with your right foot. Upon reaching peak contraction, slowly begin a controlled exhale for 7 to 12 seconds while making an *f-f-f-f* or *s-s-s-s* sound and maintaining the intensity of the contraction the entire time. Upon completion, slowly release the tension while breathing in for another 3 to 4 more seconds. Relax. Power breathe for 7 to 10 repetitions, and repeat for one more contraction with your left foot over your right ankle.

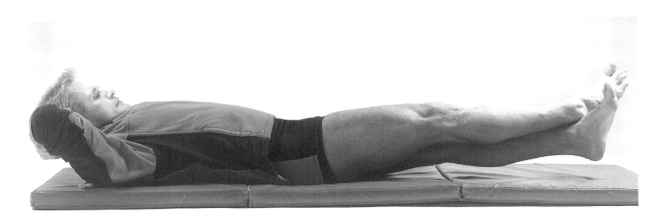

A

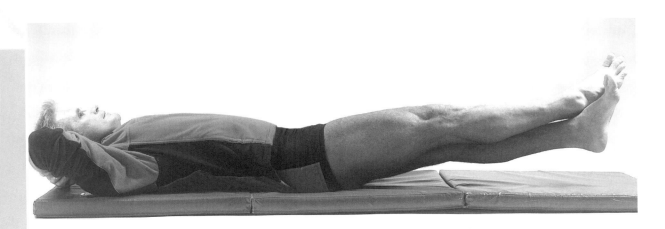

B

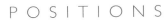

POSITIONS

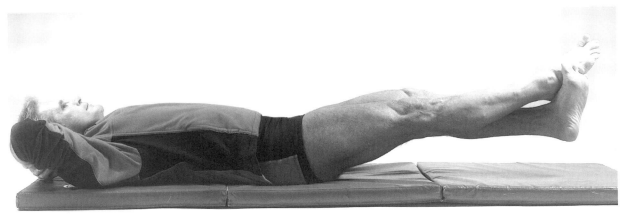

C

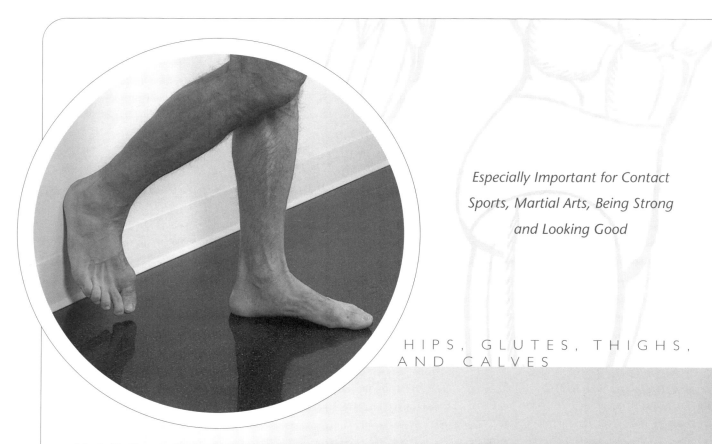

HIPS, GLUTES, THIGHS, AND CALVES
Exercise # 1

POSITION A: Start with your right side facing the wall and your feet about 12" apart. Your right foot will be about 12" from the wall. Holding your left hand on a chair for balance, place your right foot against the wall about 6" off the floor, keeping the leg straight. Now press your right foot firmly against the wall, building tension as you inhale for 3 to 4 seconds. Upon reaching peak contraction, begin a slow, controlled exhalation for 7 to 12 seconds while making an *f-f-f-f* or *s-s-s-s* sound, all the while maintaining the intensity of the muscle contraction. Slowly release tension while inhaling 3 to 4 seconds and then relax. Power breathe 7 to 10 repetitions and then repeat with the left leg.

POSITION B: Repeat the exercise above, but turn your back to the wall and place your right heel against the wall as shown. Once again follow the exact same breathing and contraction protocols as outlined in the previous exercise. Be sure to exercise both sides.

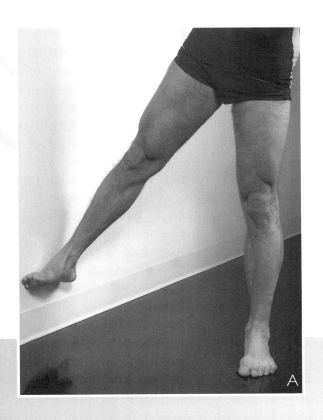

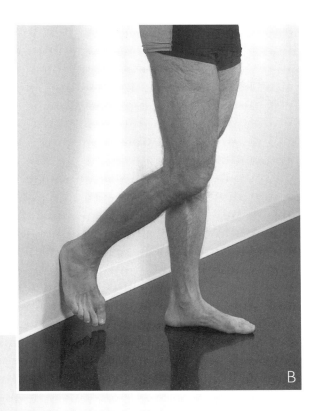

POSITION C: Repeat the exercise one final time. However, this time you will be facing the wall with the toes of your right foot making contact with the wall about 6" from the floor. Follow the same breathing and tension protocols. Relax. Power breathe and repeat with your left foot.

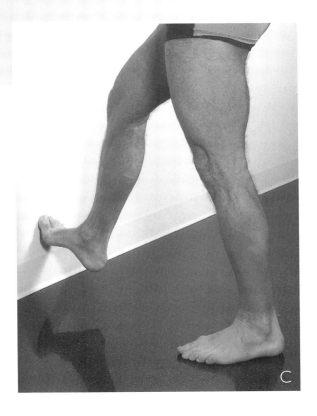

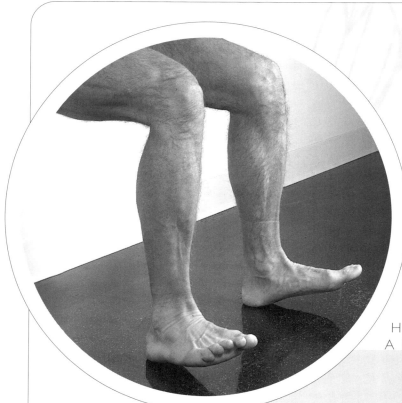

HIPS, GLUTES, THIGHS, AND CALVES
Exercise #2

POSITION A: Wall Squat (feet flat). Perform a half squat against a wall as shown. Note that your thighs are at 90°. Press your glutes and back into the wall as you press your lower legs and feet flat into the floor. Slowly build tension for 3 to 4 seconds while inhaling. Maintain peak contraction for 7 to 12 seconds while performing a slow controlled exhalation and making an *f-f-f-f* or *s-s-s-s* sound. Slowly release tension for 3 to 4 seconds while inhaling, then completely relax. Power breathe for 7 to 10 repetitions.

POSITION B: Wall Squat, Heel Press. Same position as the previous exercise except you press down powerfully with your heels while raising your toes and contracting the entire leg and hip structure as powerfully as possible for 7 to 12 seconds. Follow the same breathing and contraction protocols as outlined above. Be sure to relax as completely as possible between exercises and power breathe.

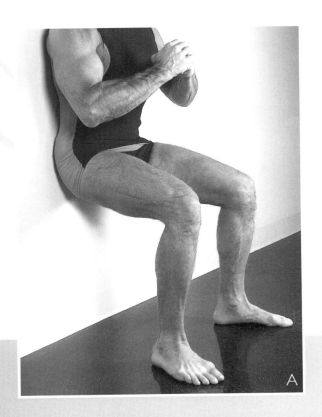

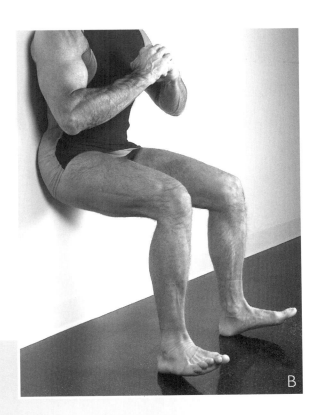

POSITION C: Wall Squat on Tiptoes. Same position as the previous two exercises. This time rise as high as possible on your tiptoes and contract the calf muscles of the lower leg as powerfully as possible in addition to the muscles of the thighs and hips. Remember to build tension for 3 to 4 seconds while inhaling. Maintain maximum contraction for 7 to 12 seconds while slowly exhaling and making an *f-f-f-f* or *s-s-s-s* sound and then slowly release tension while inhaling for 2 to 4 seconds. Completely relax and then power breathe 7 to 10 repetitions.

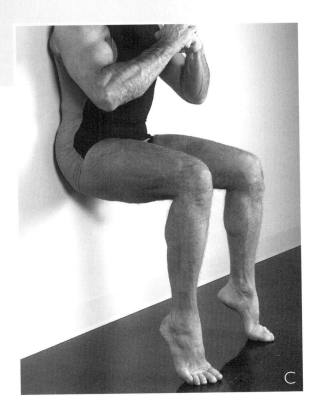

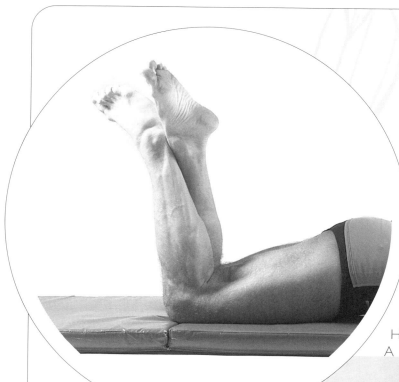

HIPS, GLUTES, THIGHS, AND CALVES
Exercise #3—Leg Curl
(to Strengthen the Muscles and Back of Thighs)

POSITION A: Lie facedown (as shown) with your feet close together and head raised, resting your weight on your hands and elbows. Place your left foot over your right ankle, keeping your feet about 3" off the floor (as shown). Pull firmly upward with the right foot, while resisting powerfully with the left foot. Slowly build tension 3 to 4 seconds while inhaling. Maintain peak contraction for 7 to 12 seconds while slowly exhaling and making an *f-f-f-f* or *s-s-s-s* sound. Slowly release tension while breathing in and then completely relax while power breathing. Switch legs and repeat.

POSITION B: Repeat the exercise above but raise your feet an additional 6" (as shown here). Follow the same breathing and contraction procedures as outlined above. Switch legs and repeat.

POSITION C: Repeat one final time but raise your feet to about a 90° angle. Follow same breathing and contraction protocols outlined above and repeat with opposite legs.

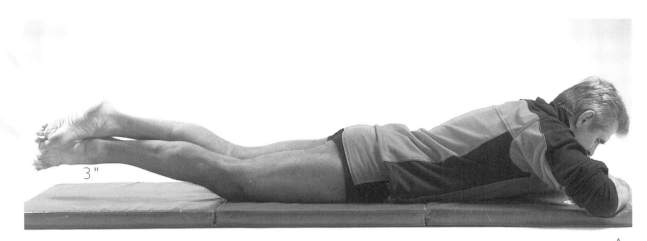

3"

A

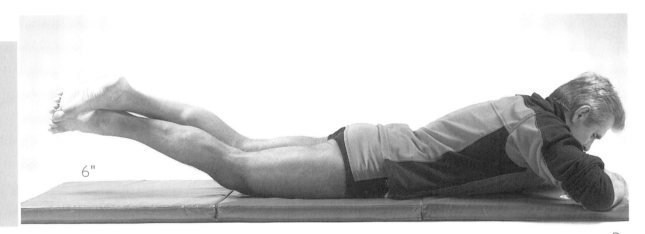

6"

B

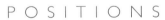

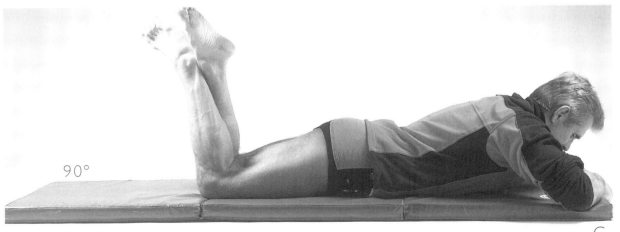

90°

C

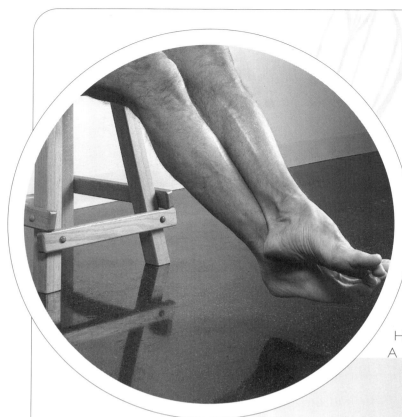

HIPS, GLUTES, THIGHS, AND CALVES
Exercise #4—Front Thigh and Knee Exercise

POSITION A: Sit in a chair with your feet close together. Grasp the sides of the chair with your hands. Place the back of your left ankle over the front of your right ankle. Raise the feet a few inches off the ground (as shown). Now push upward powerfully with the right while resisting with the left foot. Slowly build tension 3 to 4 seconds while inhaling. Maintain maximum tension for 7 to 12 seconds while slowly exhaling and making an *f-f-f-f* or *s-s-s-s* sound and then slowly release tension while inhaling for 3 to 4 seconds. Relax. Power breathe. Switch feet and continue.

POSITION B: Repeat the exercise described above with the feet raised about 6" off the floor. Follow the same procedures as outlined above for the breathing and contraction. Relax. Power breathe. Switch feet and perform once again.

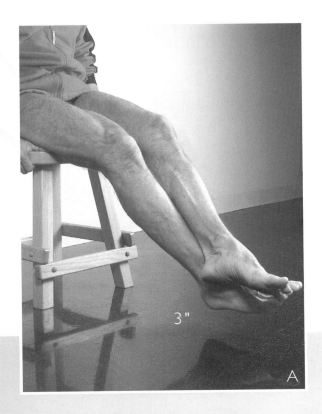

3"

A

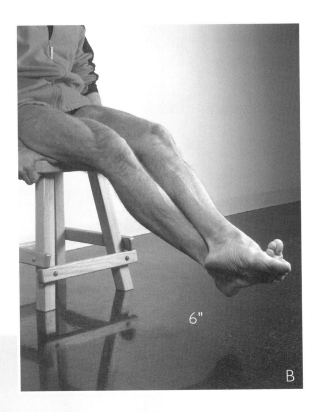

6"

B

POSITION C: Repeat the exercise one final time with the feet raised about 10" from the floor. Follow the same breathing and contraction procedures outlined above. Relax. Power breathe. Switch feet and perform one more repetition.

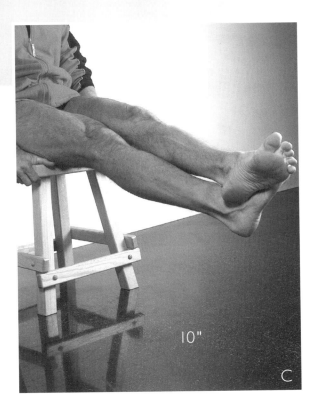

10"

C

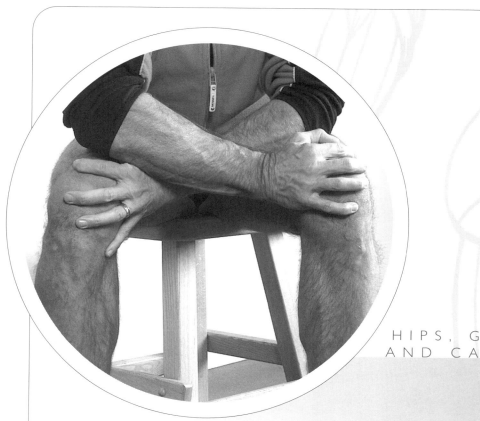

HIPS, GLUTES, THIGHS, AND CALVES
Exercise #5—Inner and Outer Thigh Exercise

POSITION A: Sit in a chair with your feet about 12" apart. Place the palms of your hands on the inside of each knee (as shown). Now slowly attempt to press your thighs together while powerfully resisting with your hands. Slowly build tension for 3 to 4 seconds while breathing in. Maintain peak contractions 7 to 12 seconds while exhaling and making an *f-f-f-f* or *s-s-s-s* sound, then slowly relax while inhaling for another 3 to 4 seconds.

POSITION B: Repeat the exercise described above. This time, however, place your palms on the outer part of each knee. Press firmly outward while observing the same breathing and contraction procedures outlined above. Relax. Power breathe.

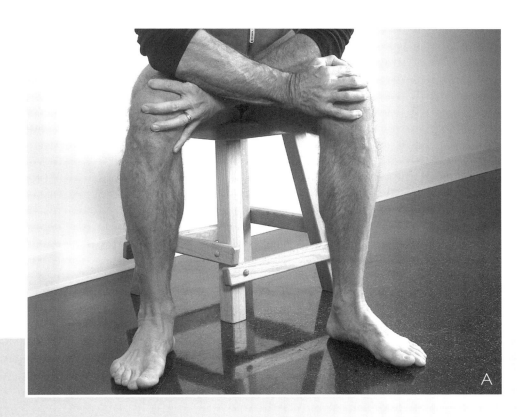

POSITIONS

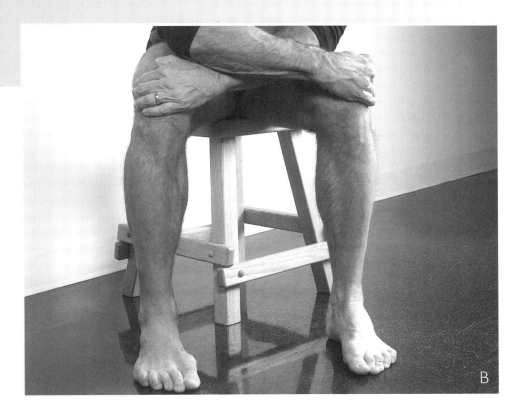

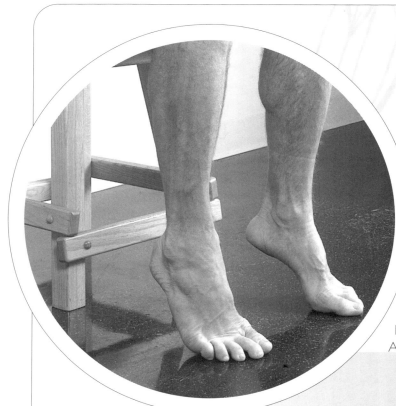

HIPS, GLUTES, THIGHS, AND CALVES
Exercise #6—3-Level Calf Raise

POSITION A: Sit on the edge of a chair with your feet about 6" apart. Place the palms of your hands on the tops of your thighs (as shown). Now push firmly up from your toes while pushing down with your hands powerfully. Slowly build tension while inhaling for 3 to 4 seconds. Maintain peak contraction for 7 to 12 seconds while slowly exhaling and making an *f-f-f-f* or *s-s-s-s* sound, then slowly release the tension as you inhale for 3 to 4 seconds. Relax.

POSITION B: Repeat the exercise described above, but raise your heels about 3" off the floor. Push up from the toes and resist with the palms of the hand. Follow the breathing and contraction procedures as outlined above.

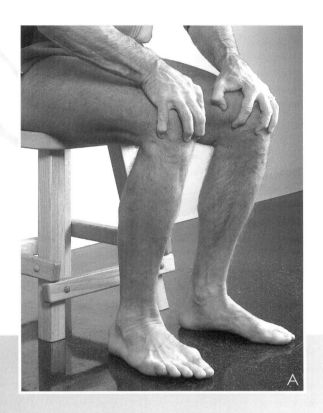

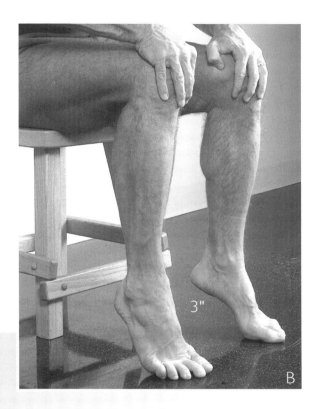

POSITION C: Repeat the above exercise one final repetition. This time raise your heels about 6" from the floor. Follow the breathing and contraction procedures from above and relax completely upon completion.

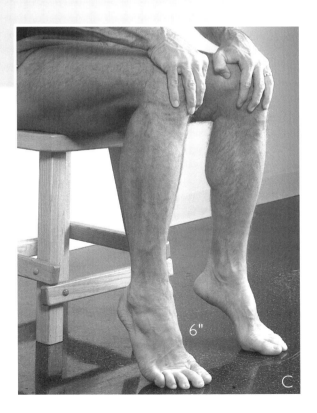

M U S T   R E A D !

HOW TO USE CLASSIC ISOMETRIC CONTRACTION TO YOUR BEST ADVANTAGE

In all there are 34 separate Classic Isometric Contractions, and in almost every case there are 3 separate positions for each contraction. This means that you have a total of over 100 Classic Isometric Contractions that you can perform to sculpt and strengthen every muscle from your neck to your toes and to do so from multiple angles for total strength development.

Now, you're probably wondering if you're supposed to perform all 100 contractions every day. Answer: NO! Not unless you're doing penance for something really bad, such as Robert De Niro had to do in the movie, *The Mission*. Then, by all means, you are allowed to torture yourself. But aside from that (and getting serious again), I don't want you to overdo it. Classic Isometric Contraction is the most direct form of muscle strengthening and body sculpting you can possibly do, and *more* is not always better.

Okay, now pay attention. It's perfectly fine to perform all 34 contractions every day as follows:

DAY 1—You will perform all 34 contractions at angle/position "A."

DAY 2—You will perform all 34 contractions at angle/position "B."

DAY 3—You will perform all 34 contractions at angle/position "C."

DAY 4—Either rest completely or begin once again at angle/position "A," and keep rotating.

Personally, I'd like to see you take at least 1 day off every 7 days. But that's up to you.

. . . .

Another way to implement these exercises is as follows:

DAY 1—Perform all 5 neck contractions, all 3 biceps and triceps contractions, and all 3 ab/oblique exercises at all 3 angles of contraction for a total of 33 contractions.

DAY 2—Perform all 4 shoulder contractions, all 3 chest (pectoral) contractions, and all 3 ab/oblique exercises at all 3 angles for a total of 30 contractions.

DAY 3—Perform both lat contractions, both spinal erector contractions (only 1 position in each of these), all 3 ab/oblique contractions, and all 6 hip, thigh, and calf contractions at all angles for a total of 35 contractions.

You can also perform the finger, wrist, and forearm exercises anytime you desire at random moments throughout the day.

And, finally, you're free to use any or all of these Classic Isometric Contractions any way you wish. For instance, you can do them throughout the entire day. In fact, that is exactly how the actor Charles Bronson, who was widely know for his incredible physique, performed his Isometric Contractions. Those who knew him well said Bronson never lifted weights but constantly performed Isometrics, and it showed.

One last thing you might want to consider is to do Classic Isometric Contractions on one day and Isometric Power Flex Contractions the next.

And what is an Isometric Power Flex?

Well, turn the page "Kemo Sabe," and you'll find out.

DAY 2 EXAMPLE

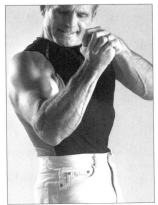
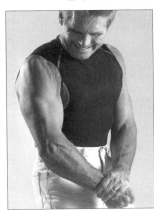
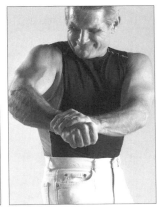
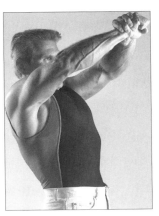

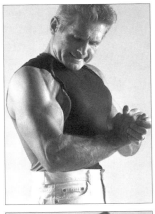
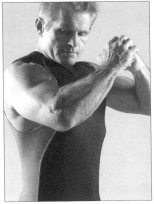
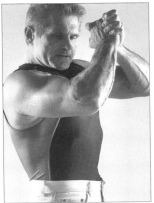

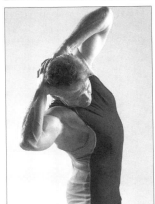
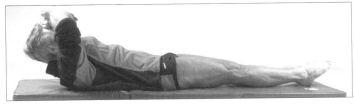
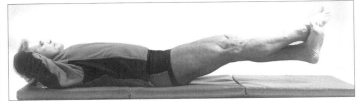

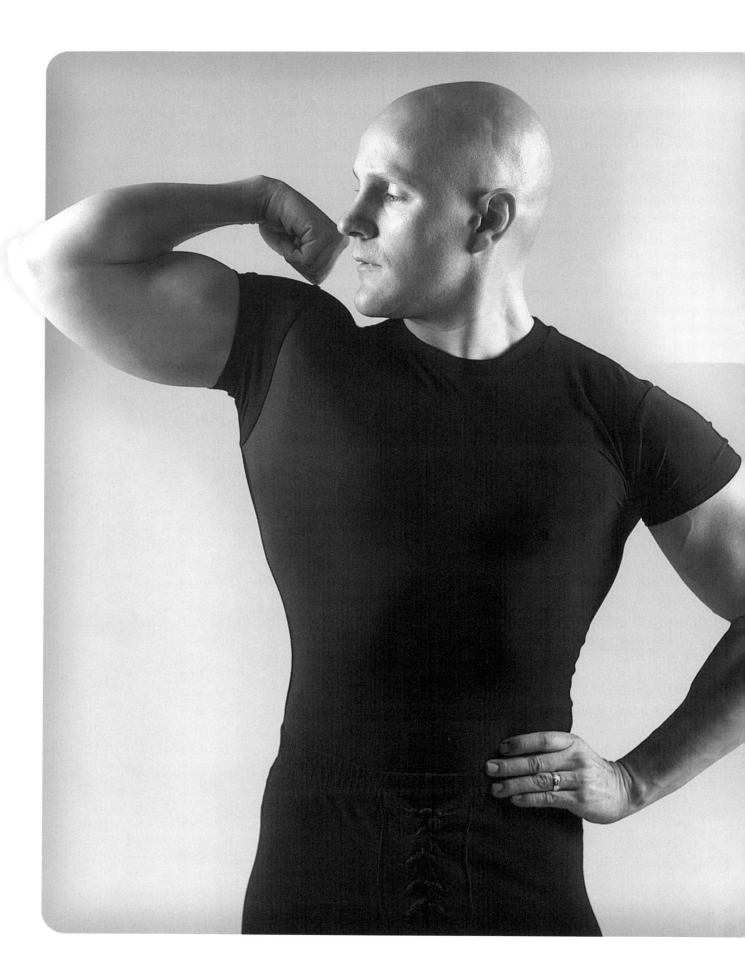

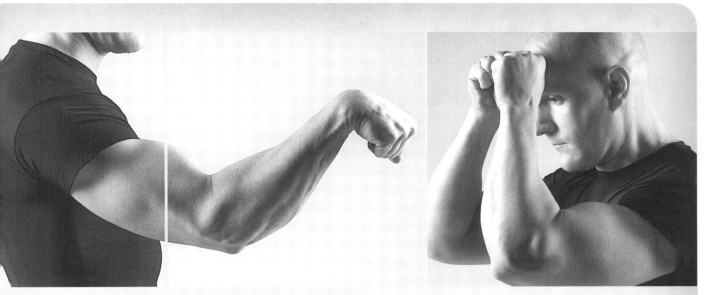

CHAPTER EIGHT

ISOMETRIC **POWER FLEXES**

*A New Twist on a Great Concept for Anytime,
Anywhere Enhanced Strength and Muscular Fitness*

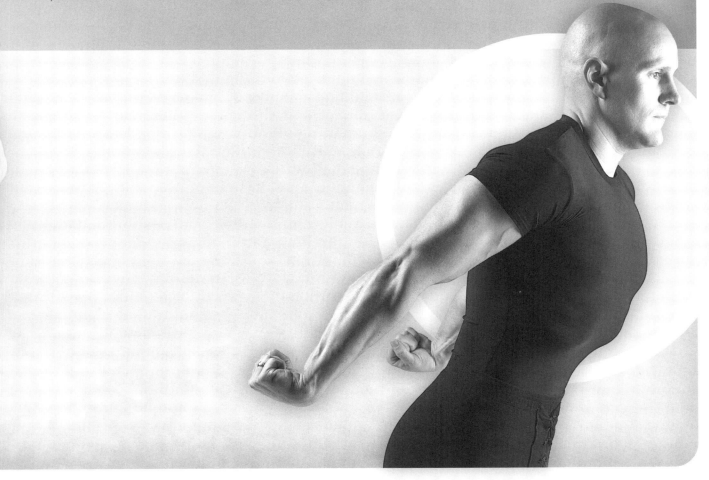

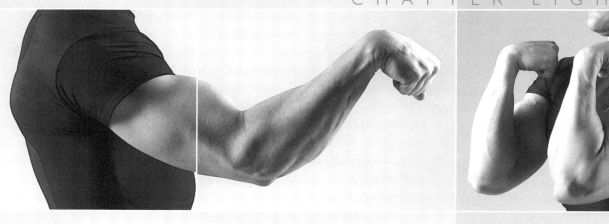

ISOMETRIC POWER FLEXES

A New Twist on a Great Concept for Anytime, Anywhere Enhanced Strength and Muscular Fitness

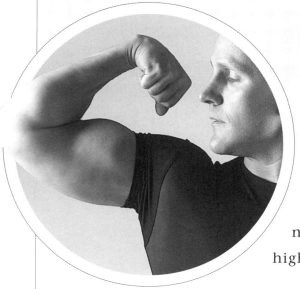

My personal history of Isometric Power Flexes begins back in the late 1960s. I had a friend named Dave Cody, who was a pushover for magazine and comic book ads that featured bodybuilding and self-defense courses that promised incredible results with little or no effort. If Dave saw it advertised, he bought it! Naturally, I had shown him all the Charles Atlas Dynamic Tension Body Building Course exercises, but to no avail. Dave's idea of training did not involve performing high numbers of push-ups, pull-ups, sit-ups, leg raises, knee bends, handstands, or the full range of Charles Atlas Dynamic Tension (DVR/DSR) exercises.

Dave wanted a bodybuilding system that required little more effort than the exertion required to send in his money order to purchase it. When I tried to convince him that hard work was required, I usually ran into circular reasoning. For instance, Dave said to me, "The only reason that Charles Atlas stuff works for you is because you're the only guy in school who can do 30 pull-ups in a row." My response was, "The only reason I can do 30 pull-ups in a row is because I'm an Atlas student." But that didn't get me anywhere with Dave. Too much time and effort was required.

So Dave sent his hard-earned cash away almost weekly. I remember one day when he was thrilled about the American Body Building Course. This course was promoted by a man named Ben Rebhuhn, who claimed on the back cover of a comic book to be "The Molder of Champions," asking young men if they wanted to be "astronaut tough." Truth to tell, it included some of the most outrageous ad copy I have ever read and some of the worst retouched photos I've ever seen.

The first piece of literature that Dave received from Mr. Rebhuhn was a physical self-assessment test to determine whether or not he needed the American Body Building Course. First on the assessment list was one-armed pull-ups. According to Rebhuhn, if a young man could not do at least three one-armed pull-ups with either arm, it indicated he had a severe weakness of the arm and

shoulder muscles and desperately needed the course to correct it. I asked Dave how many astronauts he thought there were who could do three one-armed pull-ups, but that did not deter him.

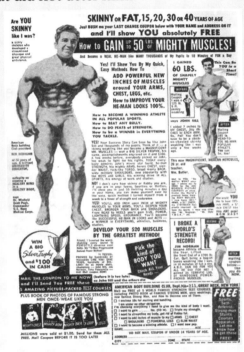

Mr. Rebhuhn then had "his mark" attempt to perform one-armed push-ups, one-legged deep knee bends, and a wrestler's bridge, in which another person was supposed to sit on the young man's chest or abdomen to determine whether or not the poor guy's neck was strong enough to survive attempting a bridge. Fortunately, the good old survival instinct kicked in for most young men, and they weren't dumb enough to even try the bridge test. Not surprisingly, Dave couldn't pass a single "test," but hardly anyone else could for that matter.

Feeling devastated by his lack of manly strength, Dave sent away for the American

Body Building Course. What he received was a recycled George F. Jowett Fulcrum Dumbbell and Barbell Course from the 1940s, which was filled with very poorly retouched photos and strong admonitions to work hard. Dave stuck with that course for about two days, then he told me *it didn't work* (meaning, *it was too much work*).

As usual, Dave dropped the American Body Building Course and marched right out again in pursuit of another course. He had purchased the Universal Body Building Course (an excellent course), "The Count Dante—Dim Mak Death Touch" Self-Defense Course (that one was a real hoot), and many others.

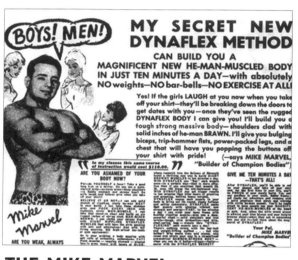

THE MIKE MARVEL DYNAFLEX COURSE

Then one day Dave told me he had found an ad for "the ultimate course," which he had ordered. A few weeks later, he showed me the "Mike Marvel Dynaflex Course." Yes, you read that right. The man called himself "Mike Marvel." In the ad, it was obvious that Mike was trying to model himself after Charles Atlas. Mike's photo showed a nicely built, muscular man with his arms crossed precisely as Charles Atlas had in so many of the Atlas ads. Mr. Marvel had a big smile and even wore a leopard print swimsuit similar to Charles Atlas.

Mike Marvel dared to call his system "Dynaflex," which sounded and read suspiciously close to "Dynamic Tension." Whereas Charles Atlas promised to make you into a new man in "as little as 20 minutes each day," Mike Marvel declared, "Dynaflex, the Proven 10-Minute-a-Day Method to a Healthier, He-Man-Muscled Body…WITHOUT STRENUOUS EXERCISE! WITHOUT WEIGHTS OR EQUIPMENT! WITHOUT STRAIN TO VITAL ORGANS!"

This time Dave was certain that he had struck pay dirt. Unfortunately, he was terribly disappointed when he tried the exercises for a week and discovered how much effort they actually required. Giving up on it, he asked me if I wanted the Dynaflex Course, and I said, "Sure. Why not?" So I took it home and read it, and I was amazed at what that 38-page booklet contained. The Dynaflex Course was the most unique variation of Isometric Contraction I had ever seen. In fact, it wasn't Isometric Contraction in the truest sense of the word, as Mr. Marvel (or whoever he really was) claimed it was.

While every other Isometric program had participants contracting one set of muscles against another or against an immovable force or object, such as a door-jamb, Dynaflex offered a subtle twist. The exercises of Dynaflex were conducted by placing the muscles in positions of peak contraction and flexing (tensing) them as hard as possible for a slow count of 5 seconds—that was unique among Isometric programs. (Why 5 seconds and not 7 to 10 seconds as all the other Isometric books and courses recommended? I haven't the slightest idea.) While a few Dynaflex exercises required minor pieces of equipment or common household objects, such as a washcloth, newspaper, or a chair, the vast majority did not require anything at all.

The Dynaflex program included exercises for every body part, beginning at the neck and working every muscle group right down to the calves in sequential order. With practice, you could perform all 34 Dynaflex contractions in about 10 minutes, if you chose to do them all at once. Unfortunately, unlike the Charles Atlas Course that featured clear photos of Mr. Atlas performing each of the exercises, the Dynaflex Course had *no* photos at all—only poorly executed line drawings illustrated the text. Of the 38 pages contained in the course, only 24 pages featured the exercises. The rest was devoted to nutrition, personal cleanliness, secrets to attracting girls, strongman stunts, and positive thinking.

Overall, this little course had some great information, and I copied it and passed it along to my uncle Milo, who also thought that Dynaflex had some unique twists he had not seen previously. Later, when I showed it to my grandfather and Uncle Wally, they both immediately said that it reminded them of the Maxalding exercises they had seen many years before. In fact, some of the exercises were identical to those taught by Maxick back around 1910.

When I practiced these exercises, I noticed they enhanced my ability to powerfully contract my muscles while performing other Isometric Contractions as well as the Dynamic Tension exercises from Charles Atlas's Course, which I would often end with an Isometric Power Flex on the last repetition. While I didn't notice an increase in muscle size as a result of performing these exercises (truthfully, I was already very well developed), I did notice a considerable increase in my muscular definition. My grandfather and Uncle Wally said the same was true of the "Maxalding Muscle Control Exercises." While these exercises helped develop an exceptional level of control to consciously contract and relax any given muscle group at will, you wouldn't develop appreciable size with this method for the same reason you could not with pure Isometric Contraction alone.

Why is this the case? As I noted previously, it is because you are not dramatically enhancing the blood supply to the working muscles, and consequently you do not achieve a significant "pump" of fresh blood into those working muscles, which is essential for increased growth and shape. Nonetheless, the 34 Isometric Power Flex exercises that I picked up from the Mike Marvel Course were really excellent and easy to incorporate throughout the entire day. Whenever I had a free moment during the day, I would perform them for 10 seconds each (I never bought into the 5-second contractions). In fact, that was one of the best things about them. They could be done anytime and anyplace, because you didn't have to resist against anything else, as was the case with other forms of true Isometric Contraction.

So I benefited a great deal from the Dynaflex Course. But that wasn't the last time I saw what I refer to as Isometric Power Flex exercises. The next time I saw them was two years later under a different name.

YOGAMETRICS
BY DR. FRANK R. YOUNG

In 1970, for my eighteenth birthday I received a book titled *Yoga for Men Only*. It was written by a chiropractor named Frank Rudolph Young. On the back cover of his book, the picture of the good doctor looked strikingly similar to Mike Marvel. When I read the book, I noticed that many of the exercises presented were identical to those in the Mike Marvel Dynaflex Course. Once again, Isometric Power Flex exercises were being presented with another twist. This time they were called "yogametrics," and instead of holding each maximum contraction for 5 seconds as the Dynaflex Course recommended, you were to hold them for just 2 seconds, then perform up to 4 repetitions of each exercise.

In addition to the exercises, there were a number of case histories about several men who had used the system for both muscular development and youthful rejuvenation. In fact, one of the case histories that I found very interesting was about a man who used the method to win a bodybuilding contest. The other thing I liked about this book was how it explained why long-term heavy weight training (either free weights or machines) would ultimately lead to chronic debilitating pain and injury. I had read much the same information in the Charles Atlas Course when I was a kid, but reading about it from a chiropractor's perspective was fascinating and made a lot of sense.

Another similarity between this book and the Dynaflex exercises of the Mike Marvel Course was that there were absolutely no photos in the book to show correct exercise positions. It only utilized crude line drawings as had been true of the Mike Marvel Course, though the drawings were different. All in all, the book had some interesting and useful information, though the exercises were certainly not part of any other yoga system I had seen. Nonetheless, I was impressed, and, as a result, I purchased four other Frank Rudolph Young titles, including *The Yogatronic Diet*, which featured an outstanding front

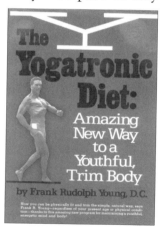

cover photo of the good doctor who was 70 years old at the time.

CHI MIND CONTROL
BY MIKE DAYTON

In the autumn of 1978, there was a new course being promoted in martial arts magazines that was written by Mike Dayton, a kung fu master. The course was called "Chi Mind Control." At first glance, the title led me to believe that this was a course about oriental mysticism and Eastern philosophy. But nothing could be further from the truth. In fact, up until that time it was the single greatest course I had read on the subject of personal self-mastery in all facets of one's life. It was well written and covered everything from nutrition, exercise, and the conservation and development of the life force energy (called "chi" in the oriental martial arts training systems) to meditation, personality self-assessment, self-control, positive thinking, and motivational psychology. It was an incredible piece of work, and it was obvious that Mr. Dayton had worked long and hard to create the preeminent course on the subject of self-mastery.

What surprised me was Dayton's use of Isometric Power Flex exercises as the foundation for lifelong strength, health, and development of the life force or "chi" energy throughout the body. He did not call them Isometric Power Flex exercises as I do. In fact, Dayton called them "chi exercises," because these exercises required a laser-like focus between mind and muscle in order to be effectively practiced. And also because these exercises did not drain one's energy reserves at all. In fact, you'd actually feel energized after a workout, which meant these exercises were not diminishing or depleting life force but increasing and building it.

As I read through the course, I pulled out my copy of the old Mike Marvel DynaFlex Course and compared them side by side. I was amazed that the exercises were virtually identical with Mr. Dayton's, including

just a few more exercises in his course. Although the exercises were virtually the same, Dayton's explanation of how to implement these exercises was the big difference. He presented these exercises in such a way that made it virtually impossible not to achieve extraordinary results throughout your entire musculature.

But in addition to the physical benefits you were certain to receive, you also developed a level of focus and concentration that carried over into other areas of your life and allowed you to attain levels of success and self-mastery you never dreamed possible. In truth, this was the "The Mother Load" that my friend David Cody had been looking for so many years before.

There was also one other feature to the "Chi Mind Control Course" that put it on a level far beyond its competitors of the time, and that was the fact it was very well illustrated with photos of Mike Dayton demonstrating each and every exercise. And to put it in simplest terms, the man was built!

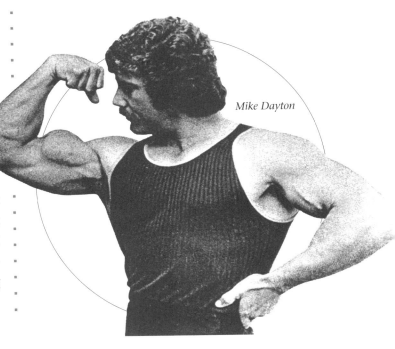

Mike Dayton

HOW TO PERFORM ISOMETRIC POWER FLEX EXERCISES FOR MAXIMUM EFFECTIVENESS

Perhaps you've glanced ahead at the Isometric Power Flex Exercises and are asking how these exercises are different from the Classic Isometric Contractions featured in Chapter 6. The primary difference between the two methods is that *Classic Isometrics* are performed at three angles within any given range of motion, (see photos to the right) and require one muscle group to resist another as you see in these three ranges of the Pectoral Contraction shown. *Isometric Power Flexes,* on the other hand, *are held in only one position* of peak contraction, where the muscle is in its shortest and most contracted state and flexed as hard as possible. Isometric Power Flexes DO NOT involve one muscle group resisting another.

For example, study the photo of the biceps contraction on the next page. Notice that the biceps is contracted to its utmost level of contraction, and it is held in this position for 7 to 12 seconds while performing a controlled exhalation during the entire time of contraction exactly as you have done in the performance of Classic Isometric Contractions.

Bodybuilders, in fact, perform Isometric Power Flex Exercises during their posing routines. And as I stated previously, it is so brutally exhausting for the bodybuilders that they have emergency medical personnel on hand at their contests just in

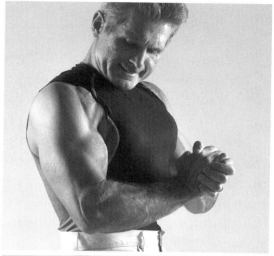

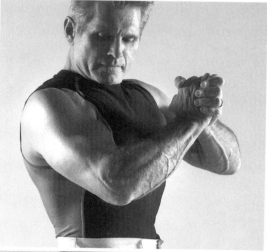

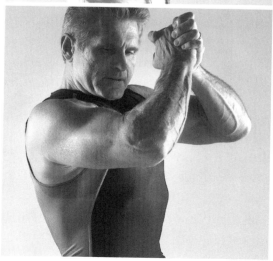

case someone suffers a stroke or heart attack while posing. No, I'm not joking!

This should automatically raise a red flag and cause you to ask, "Hey, John, if that's the case, how can performing the exercises possibly be safe?" Good question: and the answer is that bodybuilders are flexing their muscles to the utmost (just

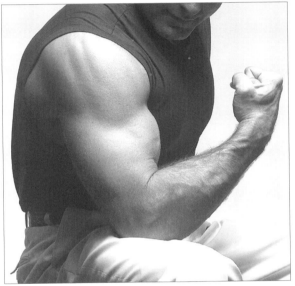

Biceps Contraction

as you will be), BUT THEY ARE HOLDING THEIR BREATH when they do so. *Never Do This!* Not now. Not ever. Doing so can cause dangerous fluctuations in blood pressure and is suicidally stupid. Believe me, physique competitors cannot possibly hold each position for a full 7 to 12 seconds while holding their breath without collapsing in a matter of minutes as a result.

Do not, under any circumstance, hold your breath. Rather, follow the same exact breathing protocols outlined for Classic Isometric Contractions. As you start each Power Flex Contraction, you will slowly increase tension for 3 to 4 seconds while inhaling. Upon reaching peak contraction, begin a slow but perfectly controlled exhalation while making an *f-f-f-f* or *s-s-s-s* sound during the entire 7 to 12 seconds that peak contraction is being held. And at that point, slowly release the contraction for another 3 to 4 seconds while inhaling. After doing so, relax completely and power breathe for 7 to 10 breaths and then begin your next contraction. The reason for the power breathing is because it will highly oxygenate the blood that is being infused into the working muscles and thus make it possible for you to contract your muscles with far greater intensity.

This brings up another very important point: the power and strength to contract your muscles with greater and greater intensity and efficiency *does not* exist in your muscles! It exists in your mind. Because of that, it is imperative that you think *into* your muscles and perform each contraction as powerfully as possible with laser-like intensity. If you do, you will be thrilled with the results. With that in mind, let's turn the page and start "Power Flexing," beginning with the neck.

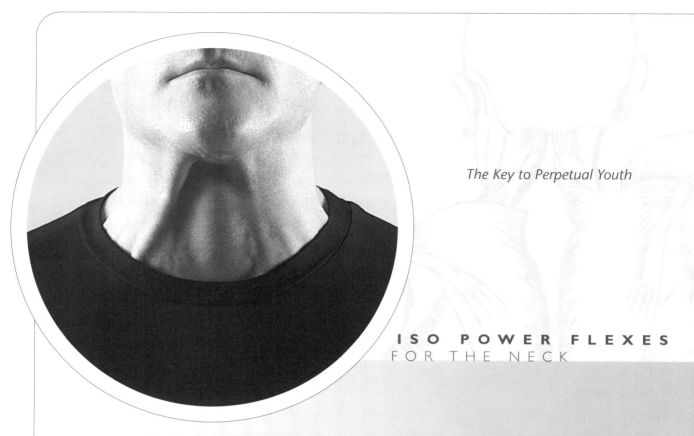

The Key to Perpetual Youth

ISO POWER FLEXES
FOR THE NECK

NECK EXERCISE #1
Tendon Flex and Stretch

A powerfully muscled neck allows you to project a strong, athletic "first impression" to everyone you meet. Male or female, a nicely sculpted neck sets you apart. And although a well muscled neck is critically important in many sports, there is a point at which a person's neck can become overly developed and detract from, rather than enhance, the overall appearance of one's physique or figure. The exercises in this section will give you a beautifully balanced neck development that will add impressiveness to all of your features.

Do not neglect these exercises. Beyond aesthetics, the muscles of the neck are important because the neck houses the center of your nervous system. These exercises also work to add strength and tone to your facial muscles. Regular performance of these exercises will prevent you from losing the shape of your face, neck, and chin due to the negative effects of gravity as you age. In other words, these exercises will help you to look youthful at any age. So let's get to them.

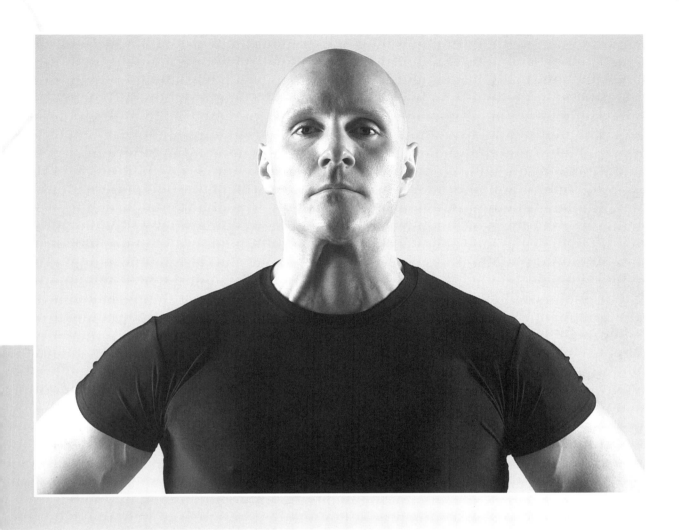

NECK POWER FLEX #1: Relax. Inhale deeply for 3 to 4 seconds while you slowly flex and stretch the tendons in your neck as hard as possible, using your lower jaw as pictured. Hold for a s-l-o-w count of 7 to 12 seconds while exhaling and making an *f-f-f-f* or *s-s-s-s* sound. Remember, you must strive to intensify the level of contraction during the entire 7 to 12 seconds that you are exhaling on this and all Isometric Power Flex Exercises. Upon completion, relax, power breathe, and then move on to exercise #2.

NOTE: **You will be following the exact same breathing, contraction, and relaxation protocols on exercises #2, 3, and 4.**

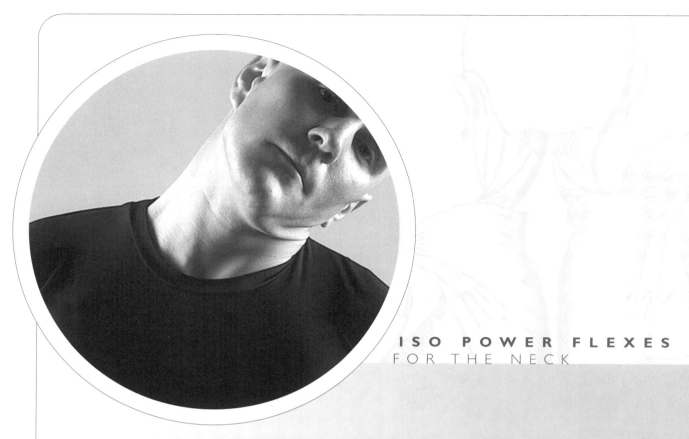

NECK EXERCISES #2–4
Neck Power Flexes #2–4

NECK POWER FLEX #2: Slowly pull your head smoothly (no jerking) as far as you can toward your right shoulder while looking straight ahead. Follow the same breathing, contraction, and relaxation protocols as in exercise #1. Repeat to left side making sure that you are looking straight ahead.

NECK POWER FLEX #3: Tilt your head back as far as you can comfortably. Follow the same breathing, contraction, and relaxation protocols as in exercises #1 & 2. Powerfully contract the neck muscles.

NECK POWER FLEX #4: Bend your head forward as far as you can comfortably while flexing the muscles under your chin. You may use your hands as in the photo. Once again, follow the same breathing, contraction, and relaxation protocols as in the previous exercises.

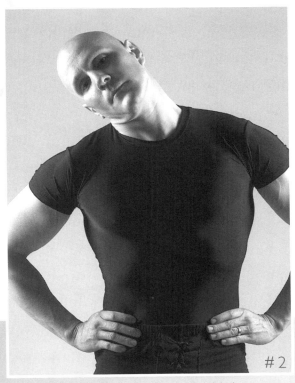

SIDE NECK PULL #2

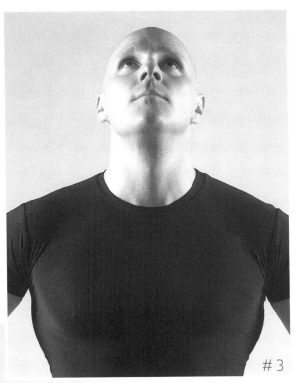

LOOKING TO HEAVEN #3

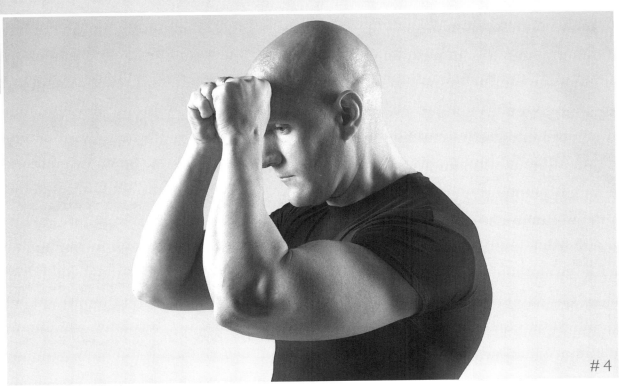

TERRA FIRMA #4

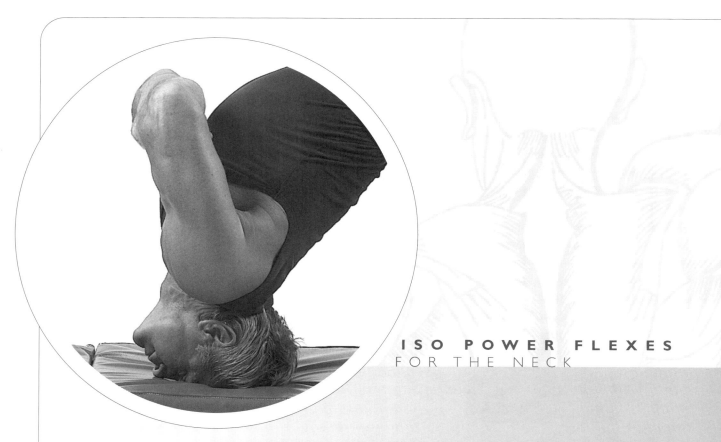

NECK EXERCISE #5

Nose-to-Mat Bridge
(the King of Isometric Power Flexes)

NECK POWER FLEX #5: While lying on your back on an exercise mat (or even a bed), slowly move into position A while inhaling for 3 to 4 seconds and then hold for a s-l-o-w count of 7 to 12 seconds while exhaling and making an *f-f-f-f* or *s-s-s-s* sound. As you become stronger, you will arch your back more and work toward touching your upper forehead. Eventually, you will reach the point in both strength and flexibility to reach position B with your nose to the mat. This is an extremely advanced exercise to be performed by athletes and physical culturists only. While you will receive incredible benefits from holding this contraction for just 7 to 12 seconds, longer contractions can be implemented of this specific exercise to great benefit. I perform this exercise in the Steve Justa "Aerobic Isometric" style for a minimum of 3 minutes each day.

Congratulations, you've just completed four (or five) powerful neck exercises for health, strength, and lifelong youthfulness.

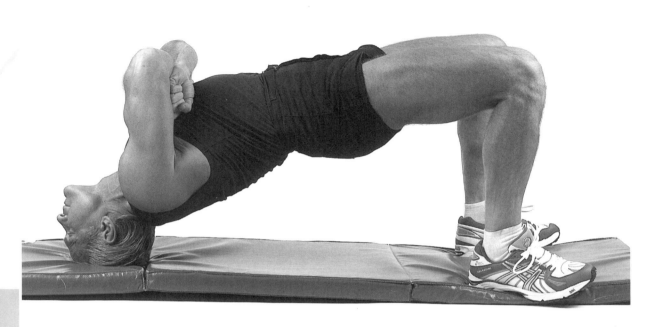

POSITIONS

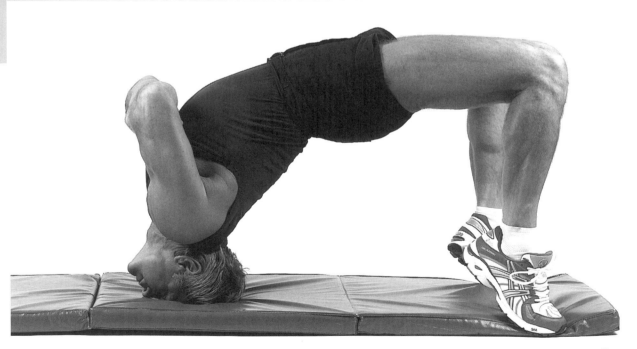

B

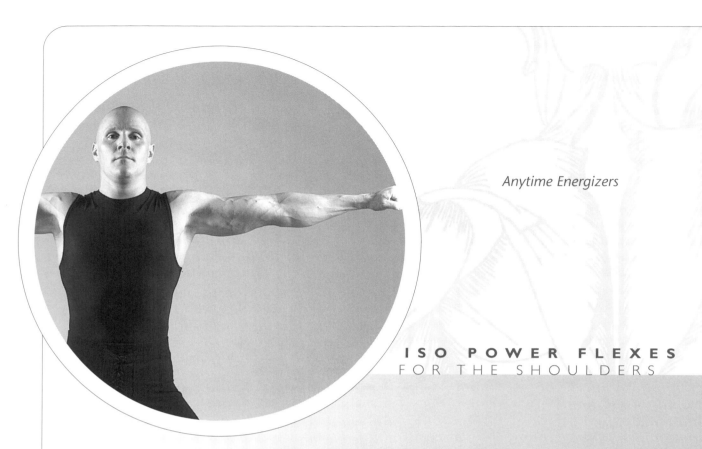

ISO POWER FLEXES
FOR THE SHOULDERS

SHOULDER EXERCISES #1–4
Deltoid Power Flexes #1–4

Powerful, beautifully sculpted shoulders project strength and youthfulness for men and women alike. In fact, several ladies have privately e-mailed me to ask how they can develop their shoulders. The muscles that we will focus on in this section are called the deltoids. When properly developed, they improve your posture dramatically, and as a result you'll walk better and look more youthful. They also make you appear taller and give you a vibrancy that improves your appearance in anything you wear. I practice these exercises at random times throughout the day. Although the movement is very short, I assure you the contraction can be incredibly tense. In all there are 4 deltoid power flex contractions with arms held straight out horizontally. **ONLY THE HAND POSITIONS CHANGE.**

DELTOID POWER FLEXES #1–4: In a standing position, raise your arms to a horizontal position and clench your fists. While inhaling for 3 to 4 seconds, slowly press your arms as far back and up as possible (your arms will elevate only slightly, if at all). Begin to slowly exhale as you maintain maximum contraction of your shoulder (deltoid) muscles for a s-l-o-w count of 7 to 12 seconds while making an *f-f-f-f* or *s-s-s-s* sound. Relax and breathe deeply before starting exercise #2 – 4. Follow the same breathing and relaxation protocols for each contraction.

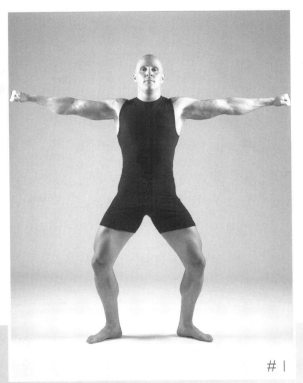

#1

HANDS IN FISTS

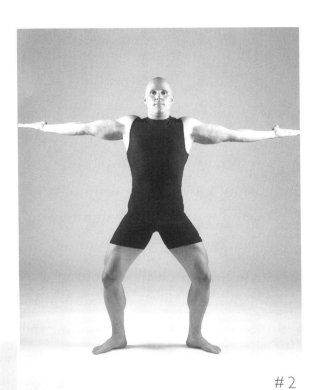

#2

PALMS UP

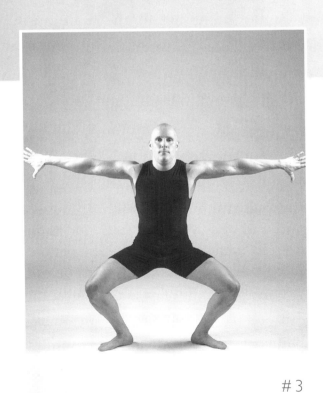

#3

PALM FACING BACK

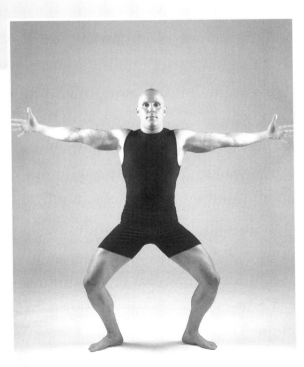

#4

PALM FACING FORWARD

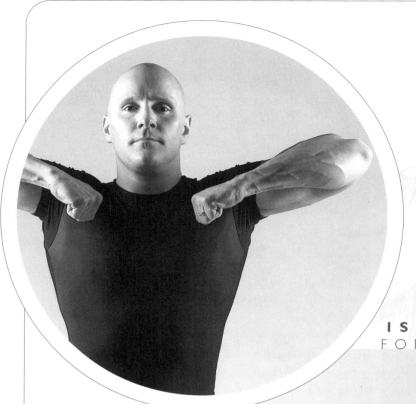

These exercises will protect your shoulders while strengthening them from multiple angles and help prevent injuries such as a "torn rotator cuff," which is often experienced as a result of bench pressing with heavy weights.

SHOULDER EXERCISES #5–6

Deltoid/Trapezius Power Flexes #5–6

As you will soon discover, both of these exercises hit the deltoids and trapezius muscles with equal intensity. This is how they are done.

DELTOID/TRAPEZIUS POWER FLEX #5: Start in a standing position as shown with your arms bent at the elbow, fists tightly clenched and held at shoulder height. Inhale deeply for 3 to 4 seconds while slowly attempting to touch your elbows over your head (no jerking). Contract as hard as possible. Begin a slow exhalation as you maintain maximum contraction of your shoulder muscles for a s-l-o-w count of 7 to 12 seconds while making an *f-f-f-f* or *s-s-s-s* sound. Relax and breathe deeply before moving to exercise #6.

DELTOID/TRAPEZIUS POWER FLEX #6: With your arms hanging straight down at your sides, slowly inhale for 3 to 4 seconds as you pull your arms and shoulders upward and slightly back. Imagine that you are pulling your trapezius up over your ears. Upon reaching maximum intensity, begin a slow controlled exhale for 7 to 12 seconds while making an *f-f-f-f* or *s-s-s-s* sound. Flex as hard as possible the entire time. Relax and power breathe before moving to the next section.

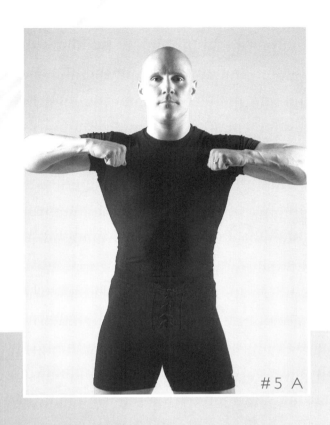

#5 A

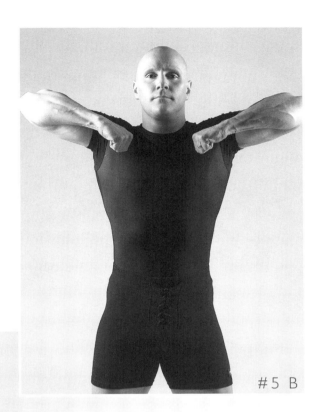

#5 B

POSITIONS

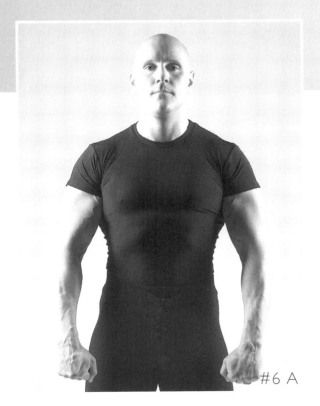

#6 A

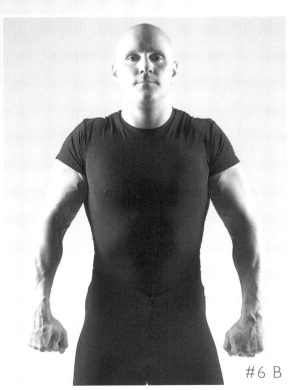

#6 B

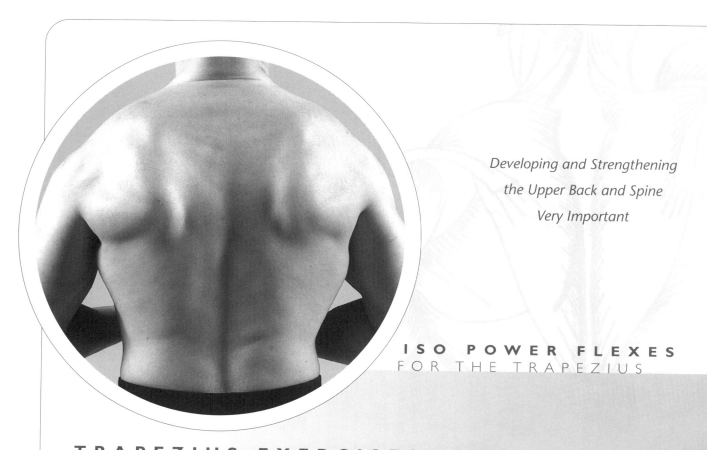

ISO POWER FLEXES
FOR THE TRAPEZIUS

TRAPEZIUS EXERCISES #1–2
Trapezius Power Flexes #1–2

Well-developed upper back muscles help to hold the shoulders back, square them off, and make them look broad. These muscles, the trapezius, lie at the base of the neck and at the top of the shoulders as well as the upper middle of the back. With proper exercise, the trapezius will help to prevent sagging, round shoulders. The key is to properly develop them but not over develop them. The following exercises are perfect for this purpose. These exercises are designed to assure a rapid response from this large muscle group with its many muscle fibers. To assure an all-around development, we will employ 4 Isometric Power Flex exercises to develop both the upper and lower trapezius muscles as well as the muscles lying directly beneath them.

TRAPEZIUS POWER FLEX #1: Stand completely relaxed, with your hands clasped together and held slightly above your waist and in front of you. Your head should be held high, looking straight ahead, and your spine erect. Inhale deeply for 3 to 4 seconds while slowly pulling down hard with your hands still clasped together and intensely contracting your upper back muscles against the pull. When your muscles start to quiver, begin exhaling

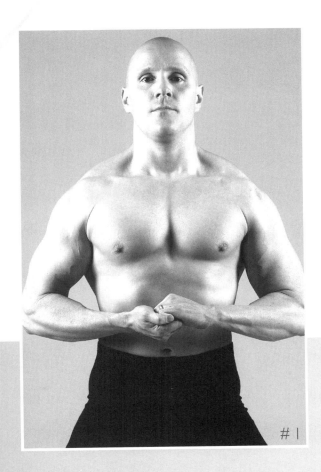

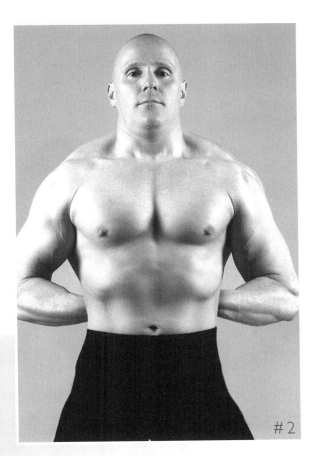

POSITIONS

as you start a s-l-o-w count of 7 to 12 seconds while maintaining maximum tension in the muscles. Relax and breathe deeply before moving to exercise #2.

TRAPEZIUS POWER FLEX #2: This exercise is very similar to exercise #1 except we grasp our hands from behind. Once again, slowly inhale for 3 to 4 seconds until you achieve peak contraction. At that point, slowly exhale while making an *f-f-f-f* or *s-s-s-s* sound for the entire duration of 7 to 12 seconds. Relax and power breathe.

Both of these Trapezius Power Flexes can be performed anytime throughout the day. I also recommend that you perform them in front of a mirror whenever possible so that you can see visual proof of the muscles contracting powerfully. You will be awed at the control you will be able to exert over these muscles.

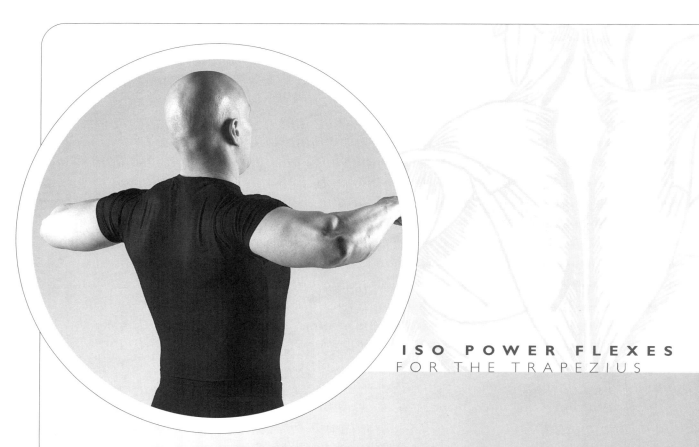

TRAPEZIUS EXERCISES #3–4
Trapezius Power Flexes #3–4

TRAPEZIUS POWER FLEX #3: With your arms bent at the elbow and held at shoulder height as shown in photos 3 A & B, begin to inhale deeply for 3 to 4 seconds as you slowly pull your elbows back and attempt to touch them together.* Pull as hard as possible and upon reaching peak contraction begin a slow controlled exhale for 7 to 12 seconds while making an *f-f-f-f* or *s-s-s-s* sound. Relax and power breathe.

TRAPEZIUS POWER FLEX #4: This exercise is very similar to exercise #3 except your arms are lowered as shown in photos 4 A & B. Once again, slowly inhale for 3 to 4 seconds while trying to touch your elbows together* until you achieve peak contraction. At that point, slowly exhale while making an *f-f-f-f* or *s-s-s-s* sound for the entire duration of 7 to 12 seconds. Relax and power breathe. As you will note, in just a few short weeks these four trapezius contractions add incredible results in both added strength and muscle control.

Don't worry if you can't touch your elbows behind your back. Trust me, I can't either. The only person I ever heard of that could was Gumby.

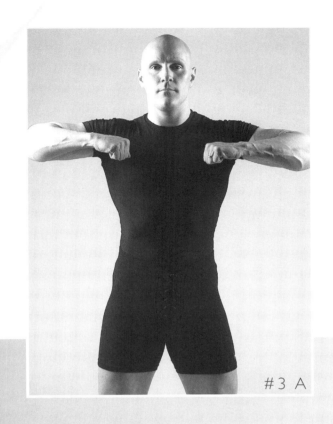

#3 A

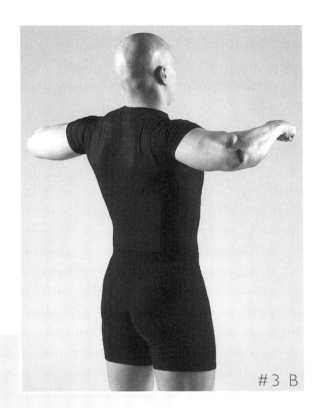

#3 B

POSITIONS

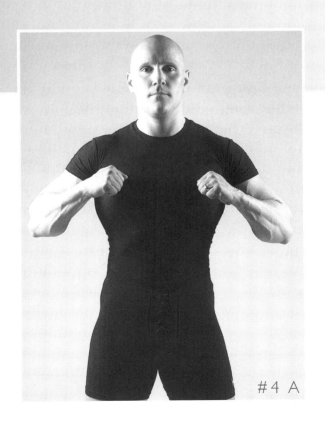

#4 A

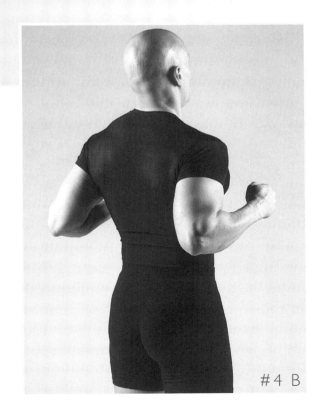

#4 B

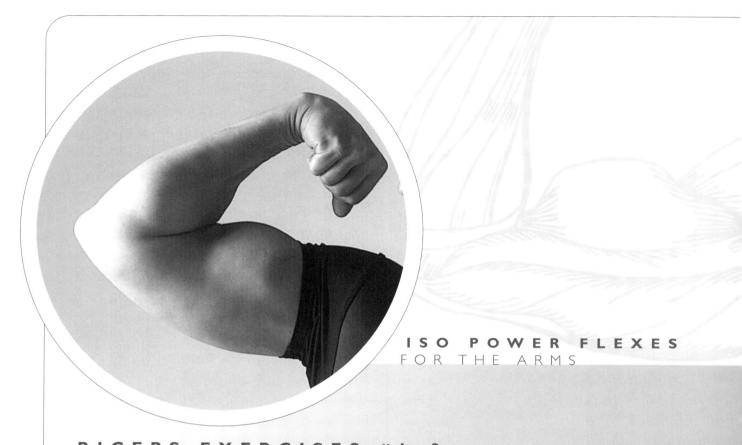

BICEPS EXERCISES #1–3
Biceps Power Flexes #1–3

Think back (for some of you, way back) to when you were a kid and the only day that you used shaving cream was on Halloween. Chances are that some other kid either challenged or dared you to "make a muscle." Do you remember what you did?

Of course, you do. You raised your arm, bent your elbow and struck the archetypal Charles Atlas Bodybuilding Pose that you had seen countless times in the ads found in the back of comic books. Even then your prepubescent biceps had a nice little bulge to them, and the message was clear: "Real Men Are Well-Armed."

Well, let's face it, you're not a kid anymore, but the message remains the same. When it comes to having a good body, well-defined arms are high on the priority list of muscles that matter to men. With that in mind, the following Isometric Power Flexes will allow you to negotiate your very own "arms deal." Seriously, if you want nice arms, these exercises deliver—big time (no pun intended). Each of the following contractions for the biceps follows the exact same breathing and relaxation protocols. Be sure to give equal attention to both arms.

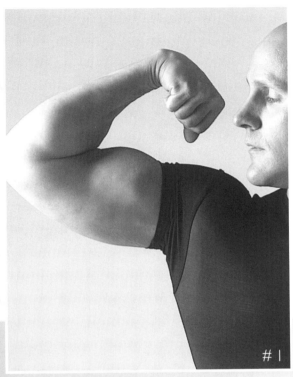

FLEX FIST BEND

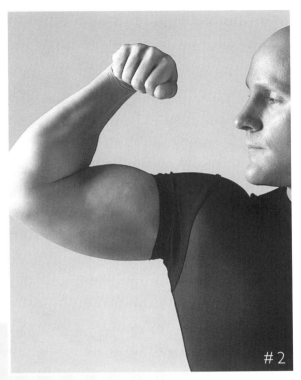

FISTS FORWARD

BICEPS POWER FLEXES #1–3: Assume the position shown in the photo. Begin tensing your right biceps with your fist curling inward as you slowly inhale for 3 to 4 seconds until you achieve peak contraction. At this point, maintain the maximum intensity of the biceps contraction and begin a slow, controlled exhalation for 7 to 12 seconds while making an *f-f-f-f* or *s-s-s-s* sound (yes, it will sound like air being released from a tire). Slowly release the contraction for 3 to 4 seconds while deeply inhaling. Relax completely and power breathe before repeating the exercise with your left biceps. Following the exact same protocols for breathing and relaxation, perform contractions #2 & 3. Be sure that both arms receive equal attention.

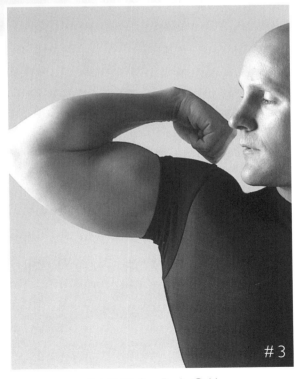

FISTS BACK

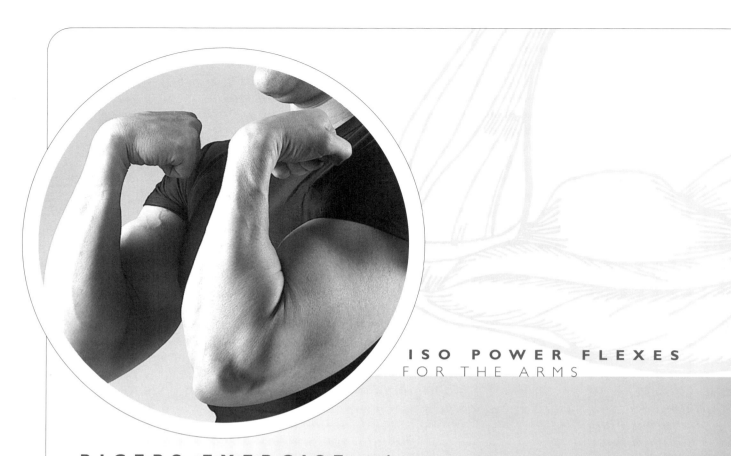

BICEPS EXERCISE #4

Forward Double Biceps

Assume the position shown in the photo. Begin tensing both biceps simultaneously with your arms in, elbows close to your body, and both wrists bent toward each other. Slowly inhale for 3 to 4 seconds while increasing tension until peak contraction is achieved. Upon achieving peak contraction, begin a slow, controlled exhalation while making an *f-f-f-f* or *s-s-s-s* sound for 7 to 12 seconds and maintaining the peak muscular contraction the entire time. Slowly release tension while inhaling deeply. Relax completely. Power breathe for 7 to 10 repetitions and then move to the triceps muscles.

POWER POINTS FOR ENHANCED RESULTS

- After performing each exercise, actually feel the muscle you have just worked—reach over with your opposite hand and feel the tenseness, strength, hardness, and density of the muscle.

- Be certain to relax the muscles completely between exertions. This is key to infusing them with the fresh highly oxygenated blood that is being delivered through your intense power breathing.

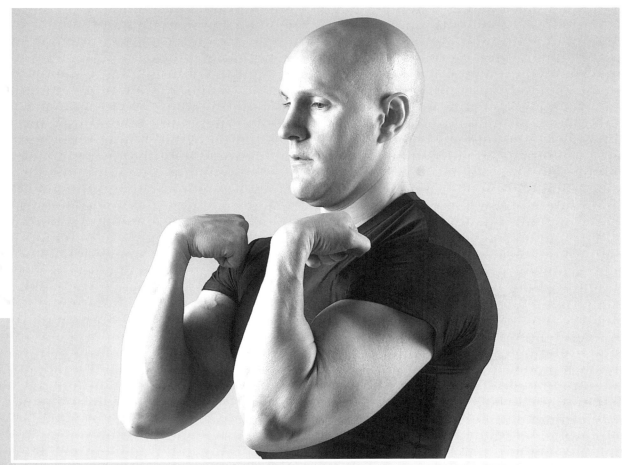

ARMS SIMULTANEOUSLY CONTRACTING IN FORWARD POSITIONS

- In time, you may wish to change all single-arm exercises and perform them simultaneously with both arms. Do not, however, do so until you have mastered your ability to both contract and relax each muscle at will.

- The positions given here are only guidelines. In time, I want you to experiment with new angles and positions and to alter any and all of these exercises to best suit your own development and muscular leverage.

- Remember to use the exact breathing protocols given because they will oxygenate your blood and amplify your results during the relaxation between exercises. Never, under any circumstances, hold your breath. Doing so will diminish the effectiveness of these exercises.

- Finally, you may notice a certain level of muscular stress and tenseness in other muscles besides those we are targeting with each exercise. This is normal and beneficial because it means that you are recruiting other supportive muscle structures that will help you to contract with greater strength and efficiency. For instance, many men notice this to be particularly true with their wrists and forearms, because these muscles are usually unworked and undeveloped. That, however, will change dramatically as a result of the Isometric Power Flexes presented here.

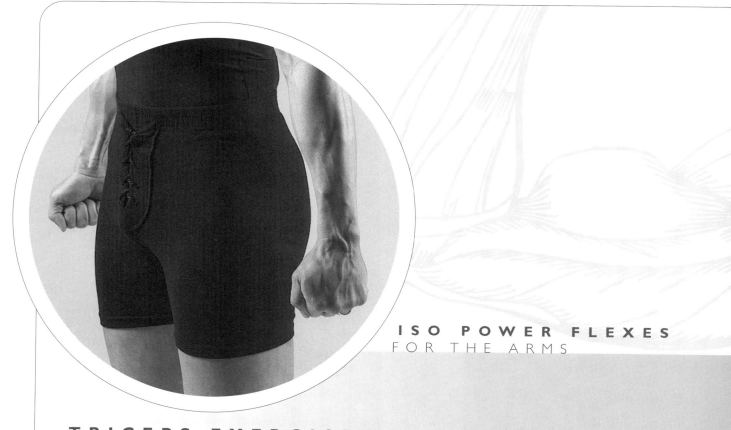

TRICEPS EXERCISE #1

Triceps Contraction, Thumbs Forward

Exercising your right to "bare arms" (how's that for a play on words?) can be extremely rewarding with Isometric Power Flex exercises because the results come very quickly. You'll notice big changes within a few weeks. But right now we need to focus on your triceps. The biceps comprises about two-fifths of your upper arm muscle mass. That means the triceps, when well developed, will account for the other three-fifths of your upper arm development.

Balanced development between biceps and triceps is essential to obtaining functional strength for sports and daily life and to be aesthetically pleasing to the eye. Pay close attention to these exercises. You will soon discover just how incredibly fast you can give yourself beautifully developed arms—front, back, and sides.

TRICEPS POWER FLEX #1: Assume the position shown in the photo. Begin by standing with your arms at your side, fists toward your body, and thumbs facing forward. Slowly inhale for 3 to 4 seconds while simultaneously attempting to bend your arms backward at the elbow, thus straightening them and powerfully contracting your triceps. Upon reaching peak contraction, begin a slow, controlled exhalation for 7 to 12 seconds while maintaining

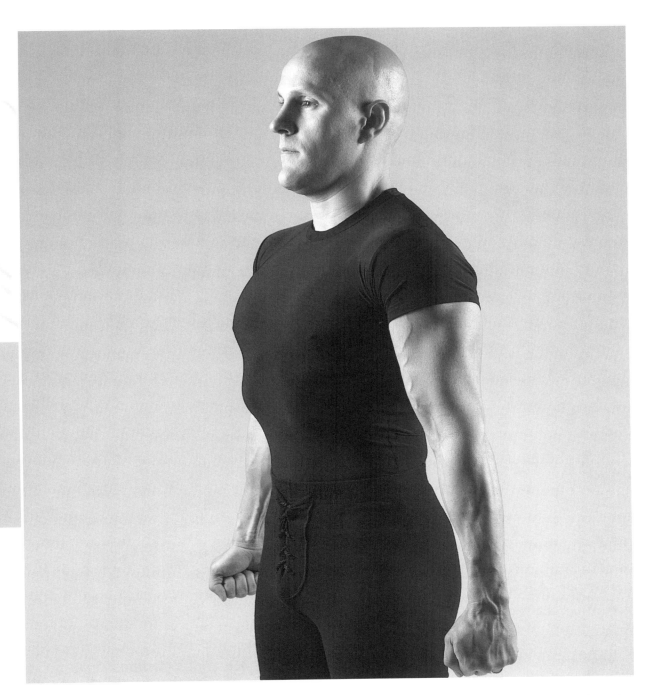

peak contraction of the triceps. *The movement is very short*, but the contraction is incredibly intense. Slowly release tension as you slowly inhale for 3 to 4 seconds. Relax completely. Power breathe as deeply as possible for 7 to 10 complete inhalations and exhalations before moving to the next exercise.

NOTE: **You will be using the exact same breathing contraction and relaxation protocols for all 5 Triceps Power Flexes.**

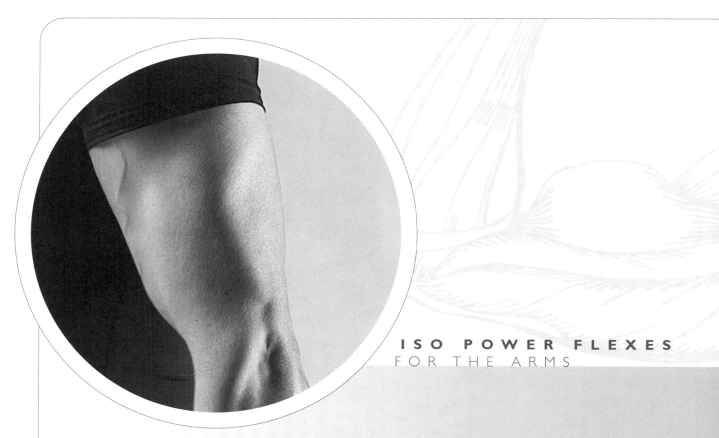

TRICEPS EXERCISES #2–3
Triceps Power Flexes #2–3

TRICEPS POWER FLEX #2: Assume the position shown in the photo. Begin by standing with your arms at your sides as in the previous exercise except that this time your fists are clenched with palms facing forward. Try bending your arms backward at the elbow to power-fully contract the triceps.

TRICEPS POWER FLEX #3: Assume the position shown in the photo. Begin by standing with your arms at your side, held away from your body with your latissimus dorsi muscles flexed (the two broad triangular muscles along the sides of your back). Your thumbs are forward with your wrists turned under toward your body. Once again try bending your lower arms backward at the elbows to maximally contract triceps.

NOTE: this exercise is every bit as good for strengthening and developing the latissimus dorsi muscles of the upper back as it is for defining your triceps muscles. It's one of Dr. Neal's favorites.

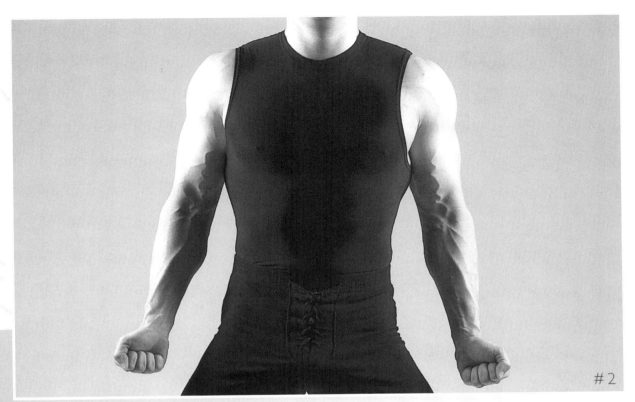

#2

FISTS FORWARD

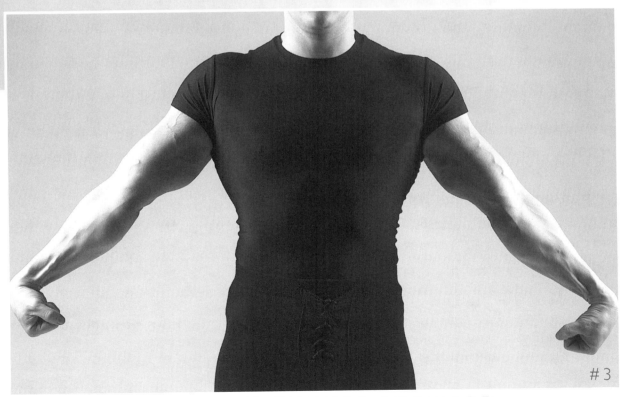

#3

ARMS OUT, THUMBS FORWARD

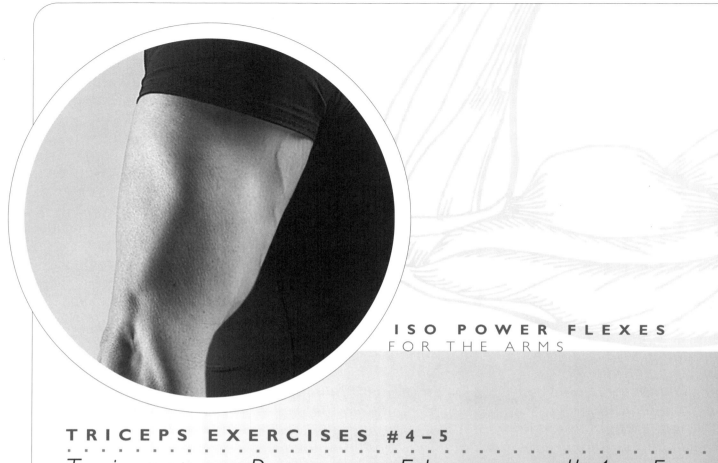

TRICEPS EXERCISES #4–5

Triceps Power Flexes #4–5

TRICEPS POWER FLEX #4: Assume the position shown in the photo. Begin by standing with your arms at your side, held away from your body with your latissimus dorsi muscles flexed, fists clenched and facing forward, and wrists flexed. Bend arms backward at elbows until peak contraction of the triceps is achieved. Once again, the latissimus dorsi muscles are as actively engaged as are the triceps muscles, making this a superb double duty exercise.

TRICEPS POWER FLEX #5: Assume the position shown in the photo. Begin with your arms held behind you, slightly bent at the waist. Curl your wrists back so that your fists are facing the ceiling. Contract as powerfully as possible.

POWER POINTS FOR ENHANCED RESULTS

- In all, there are a total of 9 Isometric Power Flexes for complete biceps/triceps development. Some of these exercises may be more beneficial to you than others. Pick those that work your muscles the best. If you have a particular problem area, such as the biceps, I advise performing all 4 biceps contractions in each workout.

- In time you may settle for just a few Isometric Power Flexes for the biceps and triceps, or you may decide to perform all 9 exercises. The choice is yours.

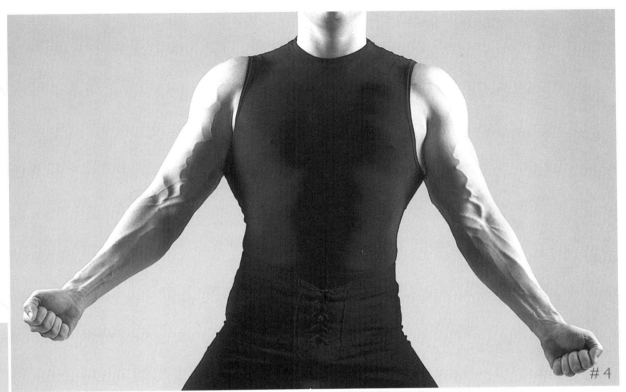

ARMS OUT, FISTS FORWARD

#4

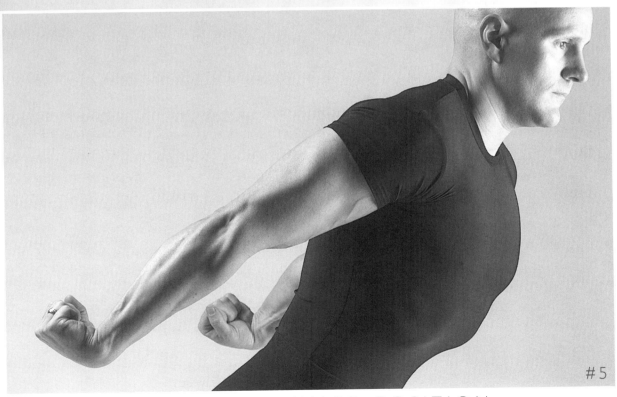

BODY IN FORWARD POSITION

#5

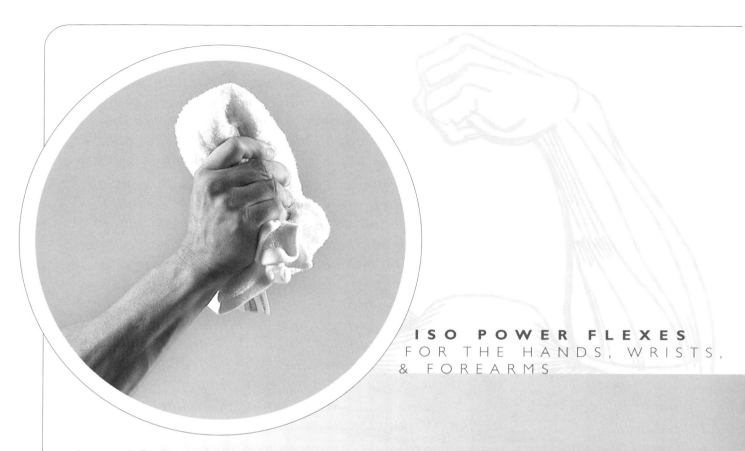

HANDS, WRISTS, & FOREARMS EXERCISE #1
Towel Squeeze

When I was a little kid recovering from the effects of polio, I spent nearly two years getting around on crutches. Because of the necessity to grip the handles tightly in an Isometric fashion, I developed such an incredible set of forearms that my friends in first and second grade started calling me "Popeye." As you might imagine, I started watching *Popeye* cartoons at every opportunity and actually forced myself to eat spinach. I wanted to be strong like him.

I even had an archenemy, the school bully, who was always kicking my crutches from under me. Naturally, my nickname for this idiot was "Bluto." If you recall the cartoons, whenever Bluto started pounding on Popeye, Popeye would grab a can of spinach and squeeze it so hard that the spinach popped out and into his mouth. Then Popeye became super humanly strong like an adrenalized berserker and proceeded to knock the stuffing out of Bluto, which is what I desperately wanted to do to the school bully. I worked as hard as I could to pop the cans of spinach, but I never quite succeeded. Nonetheless, it was a great Isometric exercise to just try with all my might.

Here's the point. Whether you enjoy racquet sports, skiing, wind surfing, martial arts, fencing, rock climbing, bowling, or fly fishing, having strong hands, a grip of steel, and powerfully

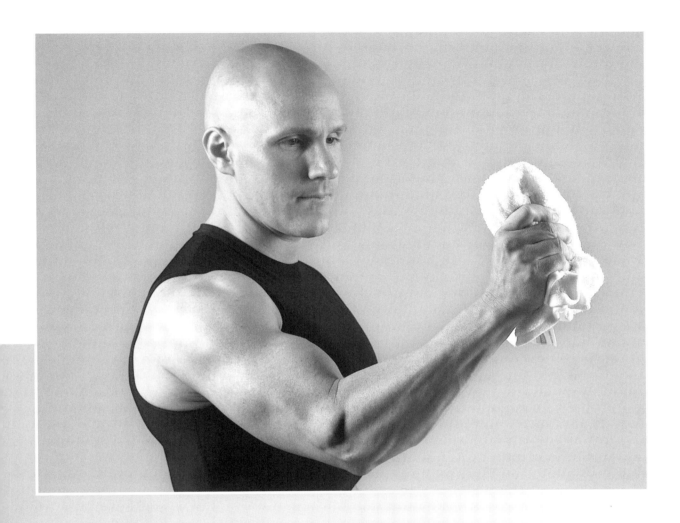

developed forearms can pay off nicely and make all those activities far more enjoyable. Although I can't guarantee that you'll end up with a pair of forearms like Popeye, I can guarantee enhanced power and sculpted forearm muscles from the following selection of Isometric Power Flexes specifically designed for hands, wrists, and forearms. And, as you can clearly see, Doc Eslinger is living proof.

FOREARM POWER FLEX #1: Assume the position shown in the photo. Please note that the towel should be wrapped very tightly and thick enough so that you can make a slight fist around it. Begin by squeezing the towel as you slowly inhale for 3 to 4 seconds until a peak contraction is achieved. Upon reaching peak contraction, begin a slow, controlled exhalation for 7 to 12 seconds while making an *f-f-f-f or s-s-s-s* sound, maintaining the peak contraction the entire time. Slowly release tension as you inhale for 3 to 4 seconds. Relax completely. Power breathe for 7 to 10 repetitions and repeat with your opposite hand before moving on to the next exercise.

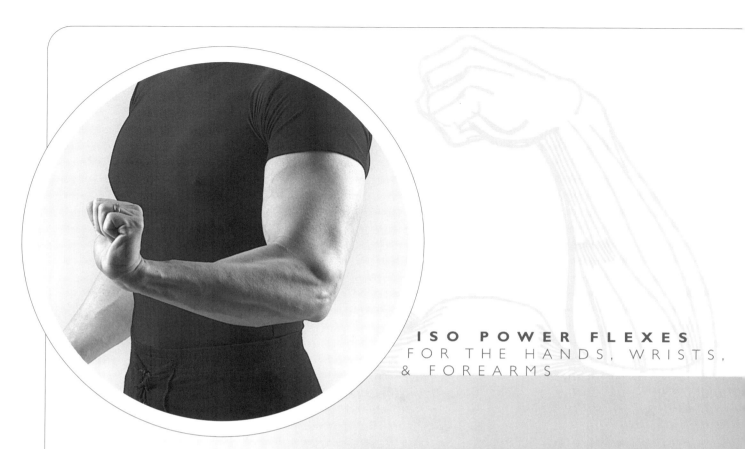

HANDS, WRISTS, & FOREARMS EXERCISES #2–4
Forearm Power Flexes #2–4

FOREARM POWER FLEX #2: Assume the position shown in the photo. As you slowly inhale for 3 to 4 seconds, bend your wrists backward and attempt to touch your knuckles to the top of your forearm. As you reach peak contraction, slowly begin a controlled exhalation for 7 to 12 seconds while trying to contract with still greater intensity for the entire time. Slowly inhale for 3 to 4 seconds while releasing the tension. Relax completely. Power breathe for 7 to 10 repetitions and repeat with the opposite arm.

FOREARM POWER FLEX #3: Assume the position shown in the photo. This is done by forming a fist with your fingers first and then flexing the wrist as shown. Follow the same breathing, contraction, and relaxation protocols as in exercise #2.

NOTE: Remember to slowly increase the intensity of the contraction in this and all the Isometric Power Flex Exercises. Never suddenly jerk into a contraction.

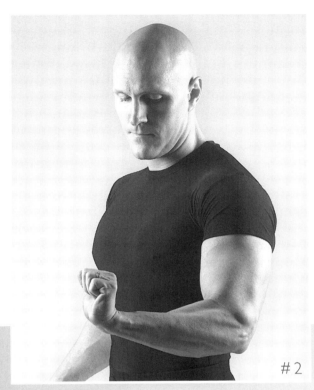

#2

WRIST FLEX BACK

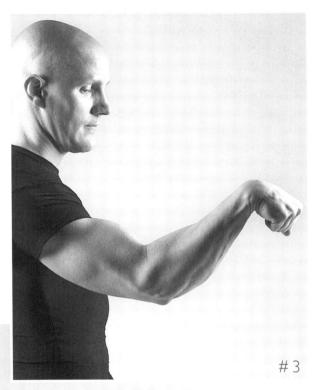

#3

FOREARM POWER FLEX

FOREARM POWER FLEX #4: Assume the position shown in the photo. Note that your fingers and thumbs are spread as far apart from each other as is possible and pressing against your upper thighs. Follow the same breathing, contraction, and relaxation protocols as in exercises #2 & 3.

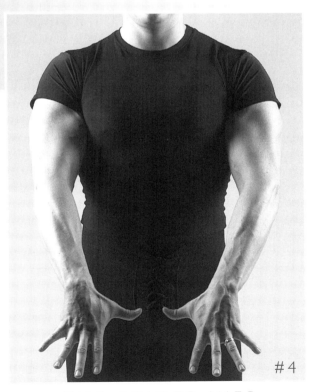

#4

THE SPIDER WEB

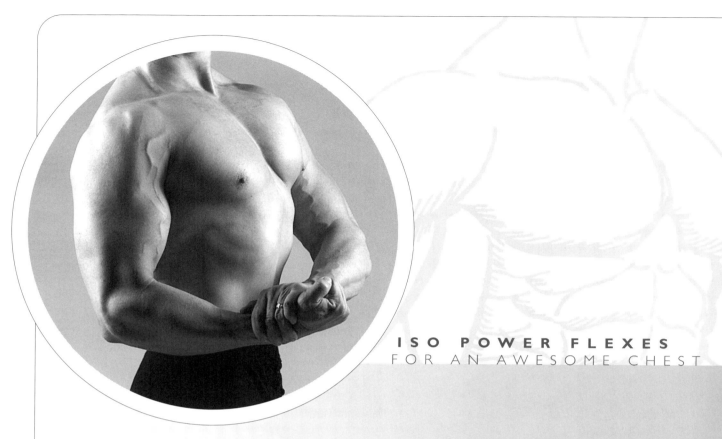

PECTORALS
Introduction

As I think back to my childhood, I remember seeing the old Charles Atlas ads not only in my superhero comic books but also in my *Boy's Life* magazine and just about every other male-oriented magazine in existence, including *Argosy, Field & Stream,* and *Sports Afield.* And why not? Charles Atlas exemplified everything that was good and right in America and was living proof of the power of the American Dream. In his ads you saw a beautifully built, healthy and happy looking man whose physique appeared possible to achieve. Even now, more than 35 years after his death in 1972, Charles Atlas's name is still synonymous with manly strength and fitness. That is an amazing legacy, especially when you contrast his image to that of the bodybuilding freaks of today who are juiced up on steroids, growth hormones, and only God knows what other chemicals.

When I was a kid, the two things that really impressed me about the Atlas ads were Mr. Atlas's perfectly developed chest muscles and his beautifully sculpted abs that looked like bands of muscle. (I was also always impressed by the fact that "Mac the Scrawny" became "Mac the Mighty" after he wrote to Charles Atlas.) I'm sure that Mr. Atlas realized it too,

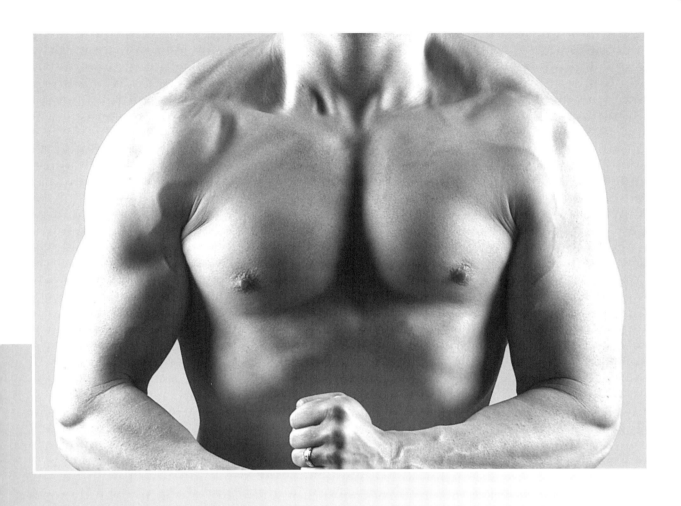

because Lesson 1 focused on creating a perfectly developed *chest* with exceptional lung capacity, Lesson 2 was on nutrition, and Lessons 3 and 4 taught you how to develop abs like Charles Atlas. Bottom line: the most eye-catching parts of his physique were the first parts that Mr. Atlas had his students develop.

With that in mind, let's take a look at the 9 Iso Power Flex Exercises to develop and define the pectoral muscles for a beautifully sculpted chest. Don't be surprised at how quickly and thoroughly these exercises work, and be forewarned that your shirts and sport coats will soon be fitting much tighter in the chest, arms, shoulders, and upper back. When that happens, don't send me the bill for your new clothes. Sorry, but that's just one of the desired side effects of these incredible exercises.

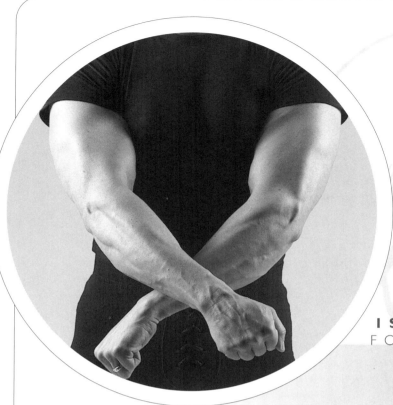

PLEASE NOTE: this first exercise is performed twice in each of 3 positions for a total of 6 Iso Power Flex Contractions. The reason for this is so that each arm occupies both top and bottom positions.

ISO POWER FLEXES
FOR AN AWESOME CHEST

PECTORAL EXERCISES #1–6
Pectoral Power Flexes #1–6

POSITION A (POWER FLEXES 1 & 2): While inhaling deeply for 3 to 4 seconds, cross your right arm over your left arm just below your elbows and straight down in front of your body close to your waistline. You must twist your arms so that your fists are facing each other and your thumbs are turned downward (clockwise for your left arm and counterclockwise for your right arm). Twist your arms as intensely as possible, thereby contracting your shoulder, arm, forearm, and especially your chest muscles. Flex as hard as possible as you slowly exhale for 7 to 12 seconds while making an *f-f-f-f* or *s-s-s-s* sound. Upon completion, relax. Power breathe for 7 to 10 breaths, and **THEN REPEAT THIS SAME EXERCISE WITH THE LEFT ARM OVER THE RIGHT.** Follow the same protocols for contraction and relaxation. Power breathe for another 7 to 10 breaths before moving to position B for contractions 3 and 4.

POSITION B (POWER FLEXES 3 & 4): Your arms are crossed exactly as in position A. This time your arms are held straight out from your body at shoulder level. Follow the same breathing and relaxing protocols as in position A. **BE SURE TO REPEAT WITH LEFT SIDE.**

POSITION C (POWER FLEXES 5 & 6): Once again, your arms are crossed exactly as in the two preceding positions with your arms held pointing up at eye level. Follow the same

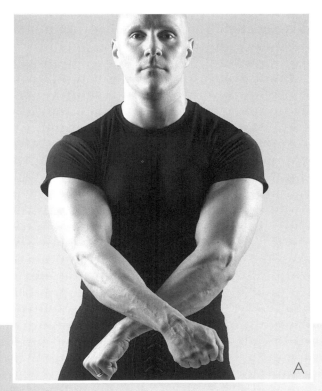

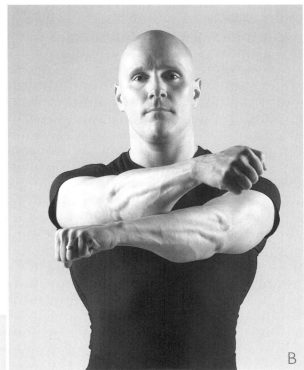

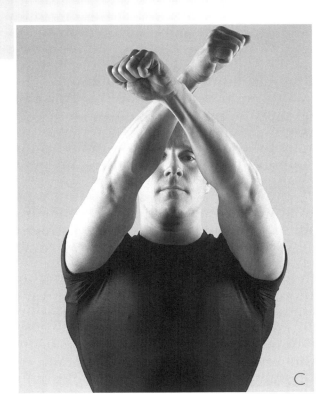

breathing and relaxing protocols as in position A & B. **BE SURE TO REPEAT WITH LEFT ARM IN TOP POSITION.**

NOTE: these 6 positions create very powerful and intense contractions of the pectoral muscles and may cause the muscles to cramp. If that happens, simply relax the muscle and rub gently until the cramp subsides. In just a few weeks you'll be amazed at the shape and definition of your pectoral muscles, particularly if you practice these 6 contractions in combination with the Classic Isometric Contractions for the pectoral muscles as found in Chapter 6.

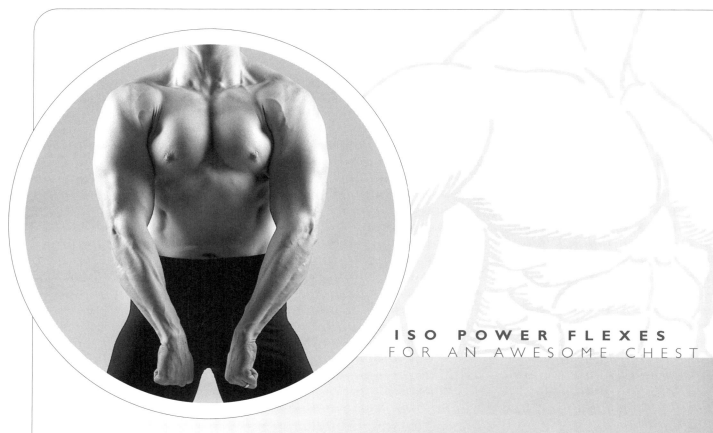

PECTORAL EXERCISES #7–9
Pectoral Power Flexes #7–9

PECTORAL POWER FLEX #7—THE MCSWEENEY WRIST TWIST

This exercise is the starting position of a DVR (Dynamic Visualized Resistance) exercise that was taught by the famous martial arts Master John McSweeney. It allows you to powerfully contract both triceps and pectorals simultaneously.

With the back of your hands together as shown and your arms held straight down in front of your body, pull down as hard and intensely as possible while inhaling for 3 to 4 seconds. Imagine that your arms are pulling your shoulders together and over the front of your body. Upon reaching peak contraction, begin a slow, controlled exhalation for 7 to 12 seconds while making an *f-f-f-f* or *s-s-s-s* sound—contracting as powerfully as possible the entire time. Relax and power breathe for 7 to 10 breaths before moving to contraction #8.

PECTORAL POWER FLEX #8—FOR THE SERRATUS MAGNUS OR RIB BOX

Assume the position shown with your shoulders back and down. Your hands are flat and open on your abdomen. While inhaling for 3 to 4 seconds, expand your rib cage as far as possible, attempting to push out the air and spread your rib cage. Upon reaching peak contraction, begin a slow, perfectly controlled exhalation for 7 to 12 seconds while making an *f-f-f-f* or *s-s-s-s* sound—trying to maintain the flexion of your rib cage to its maximum. Relax and power breathe.

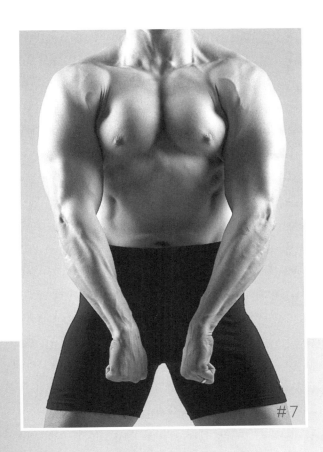

#7

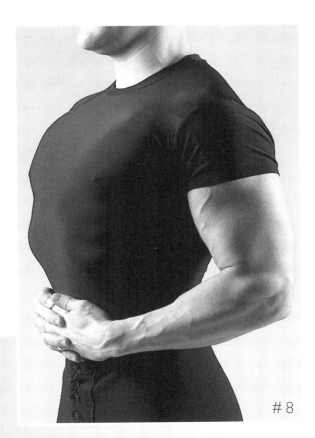

#8

PECTORAL POWER FLEX #9—(NO PHOTO SHOWN OR NECESSARY)

I learned this exercise from the original Charles Atlas Course and have been practicing it since I was 10 years old. Though it is very simple and can be done anytime during the day, it yields great results and enhanced muscle control.

While standing erect with your hands hanging normally at your sides, inhale for 3 to 4 seconds while bearing down the shoulders and arms at the same time, thereby contracting the chest muscles as powerfully as possible. Upon reaching peak contraction, begin to slowly exhale for 7 to 12 seconds while making an *f-f-f-f* or *s-s-s-s* sound. Relax and power breathe.

So there you have it, 9 powerful contractions that will shape and enhance the strength of your pectoral muscles in the most direct manner possible. In addition, you may perform the Classic Isometric Contractions from Chapter 6 to achieve the best, most enhanced results.

One other exercise you may wish to add to your chest building program is the Atlas Push-up Variation #1, which is found on page 97. This exercise was number one in the world famous Charles Atlas Dynamic Tension Bodybuilding Course and was foundational, because of the incredible blood volume that it pumps into the muscles. Believe me, you'll know what the word *pump* means after you've done a few sets of it.

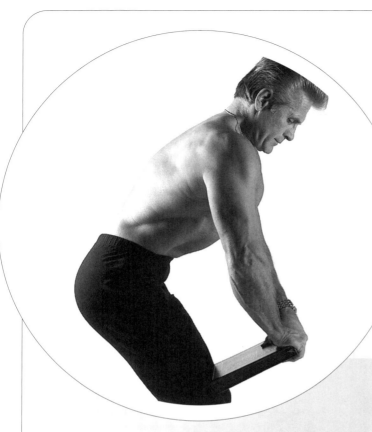

LATS EXERCISE #1

Latissimus Dorsi Flex #1

Back in the history section, I shared with you the page from Victor Hugo's *Les Misérables* that told how Jean Valjean had used a mysterious system of "statics" to develop his incredible strength and physique. Well, the story didn't end there. As a result of his incredible development due to his daily bouts with "Static Isometric Contraction," Valjean had a perfect "V" shaped back. It was so perfect that Inspector Javert could pick him out in a crowd. So, the bottom line is that I will now show you a mysterious system of 3 statics that are guaranteed to develop awesome "lats," and if Javert comes after you, don't blame me.

LATISSIMUS POWER FLEX #1: Position a book just above the top of your knee as shown. Inhale deeply for 3 to 4 seconds while pulling down and contracting your latissimus dorsi muscles as powerfully as possible. Upon reaching peak contraction, begin a slow, controlled exhalation for 7 to 12 seconds while making an *f-f-f-f* or *s-s-s-s* sound. Upon completion, relax and power breathe for 7 to 10 breaths.

This is my favorite Latissimus Power Flex exercise. It yields excellent results.

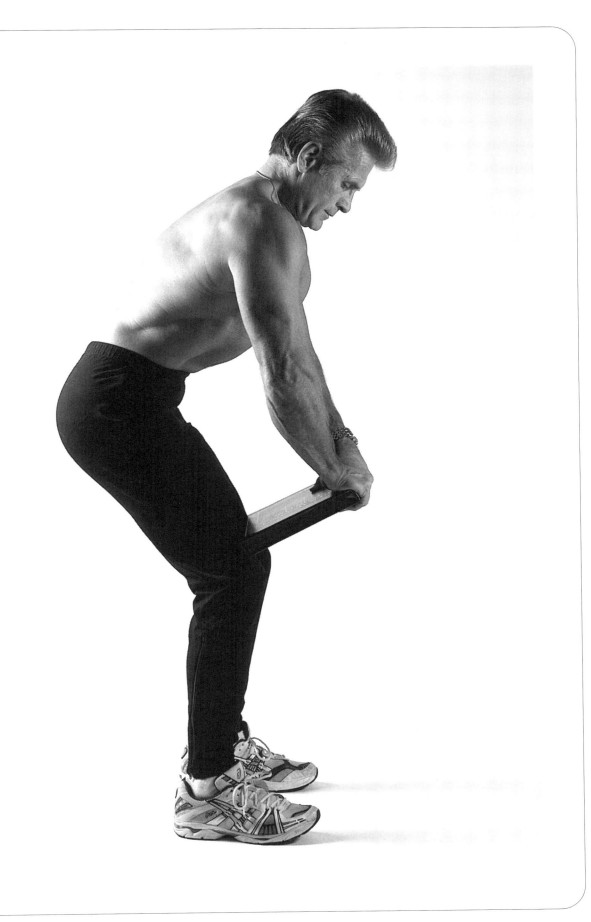

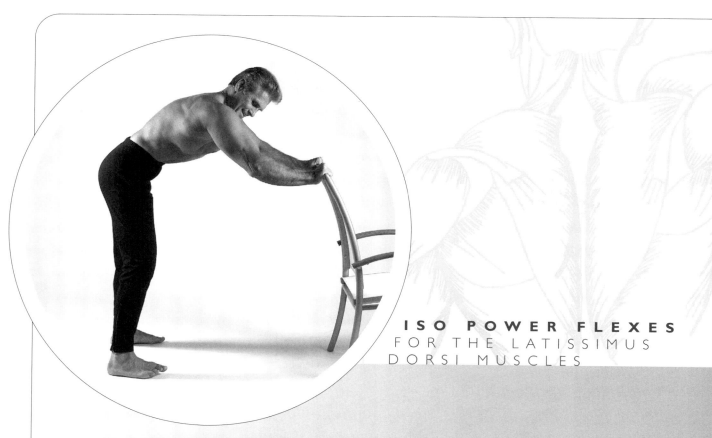

ISO POWER FLEXES
FOR THE LATISSIMUS DORSI MUSCLES

LATS EXERCISES #2–3

Latissimus Dorsi Flexes #2–3

LATISSIMUS POWER FLEX #2: Using the back of a chair, reach out and grasp the top of it. Keep your back as straight as possible and keep your shoulders stationary as you inhale for 3 to 4 seconds while tensing your back muscles as powerfully as possible. Upon reaching peak contraction, begin a slow, controlled exhalation for 7 to 12 seconds while making an *f-f-f-f* or *s-s-s-s* sound. Upon completion, relax and power breathe for 7 to 10 breaths before moving to contraction #3.

LATISSIMUS POWER FLEX #3: Standing in front of a mirror, flex you lats out as far as possible while deeply inhaling for 3 to 4 seconds. Watch the muscles closely, and upon reaching peak contraction, begin a slow, controlled exhalation for 7 to 12 seconds while making an *f-f-f-f* or *s-s-s-s* sound. Upon completion, relax and power breathe for 7 to 10 breaths before moving to the next section.

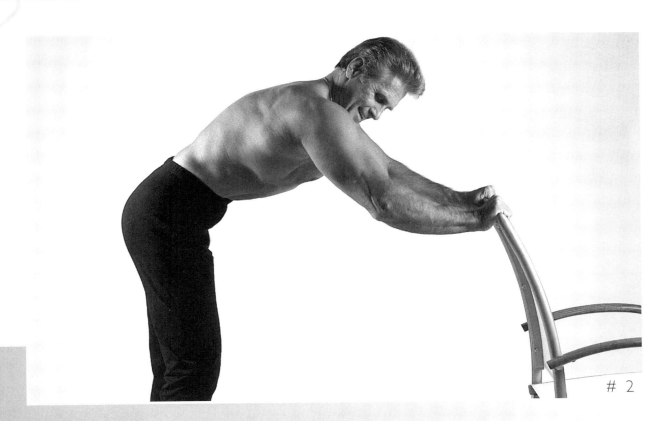

2

POSITIONS

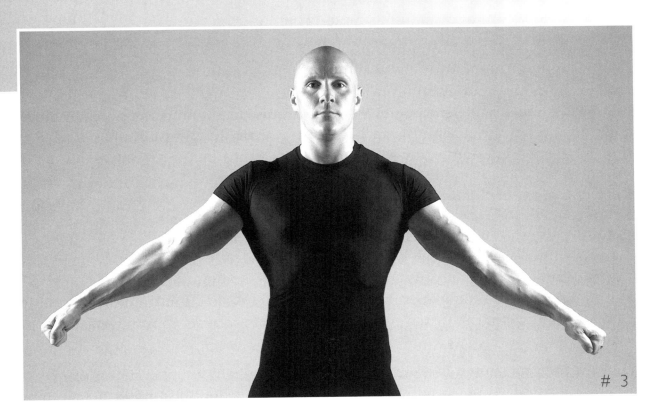

3

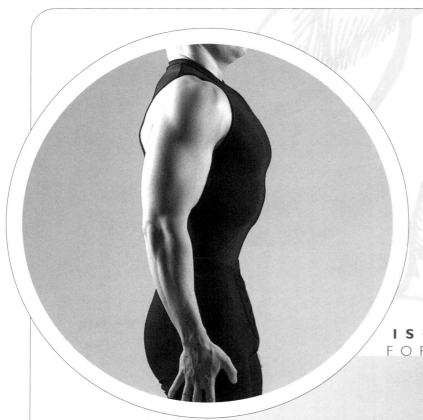

"The abdomen is the reason why man does not easily take himself for a god." —Friedrich Nietzsche

ISO POWER FLEXES
FOR THE ABDOMINALS

ABS EXERCISE #1
. . . .
Abdominal Contraction #1

Let's be real. No muscle group has received as much attention from the general public in the last few years as has the abdominals. In fact, if you turn on the television and start channel surfing, I can almost guarantee you will find one or more infomercials trying to sell you the latest ab gizmo. But the truth is *you don't need any of them.* If you perform Isometric Contraction of the abdominal muscles multiple times throughout the day, you will do far more for your abs and waistline than any ab gizmo could ever accomplish. How so? Because with Isometric Power Flex Contraction you are exercising the abdominal muscle structure in the *most direct way possible;* whereas, if you are using any ab gizmo, you'll be working against "it" rather than focusing your attention on the contraction of the abdominal muscles themselves. As a result, you'll be spending money you don't need to spend and still not get the results you want and can easily achieve by learning how to contract your abdominal muscles directly the Iso Power Flex way.

And by the way, no amount of exercise will give you beautifully sculpted abdominals if they are hidden under a layer of fat. To get rid of that layer of fat, follow the nutritional suggestions

ABS POWER FLEX #1: At any time throughout your day, while either sitting or standing, simply inhale for 3 to 4 seconds while trying to touch the front abdominal muscles to the spine (at least that's how it feels). While maintaining the contraction, slowly exhale for 7 to 12 seconds while making an *f-f-f-f* or *s-s-s-s* sound. Upon completion, relax and power breathe for 7 to 10 breaths.

This exercise can be repeated throughout the day with fantastic results. So now you have no reason to ever have a bulging gut—not now . . . not ever.

outlined earlier and add 20 minutes of daily aerobic/cardio exercise to burn calories and increase your basal metabolic rate.

So let's get to the 5 abdominal Iso Power Flexes. The last 4 are done in sequence, and #1 can be done anytime throughout the day to flatten the abdomen to an amazing extent.

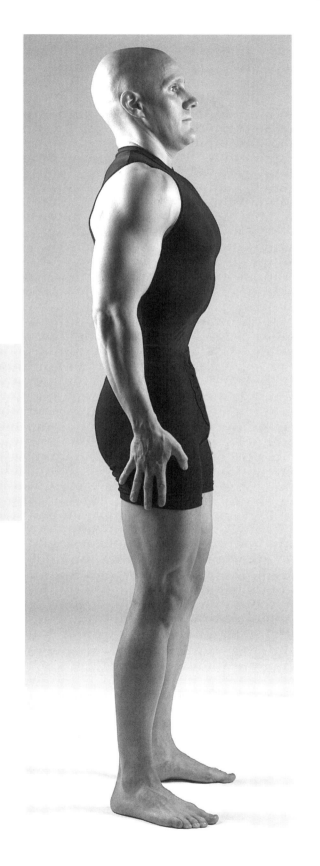

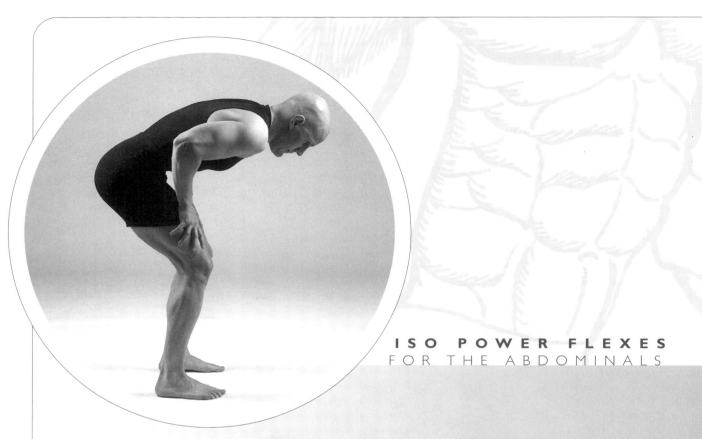

ABS EXERCISES #2–5
Abdominal Contractions #2–5

ABS POWER FLEXES #2–5: Study the photos and note the 4 positions. Starting with position A, you complete each position following the exact same contraction and relaxation protocols.

Inhale deeply for 3 to 4 seconds while bending slightly forward with your hands on your thighs and flexing your abdominals downward as powerfully as possible into a peak contraction. Slowly exhale for 7 to 12 seconds while making an *f-f-f-f* or *s-s-s-s* sound. Upon completion, relax and power breathe for 7 to 10 breaths.

Continue with positions B, C, and D.

Although you can perform multiple repetitions of each position throughout the day, only one is necessary to achieve excellent results.

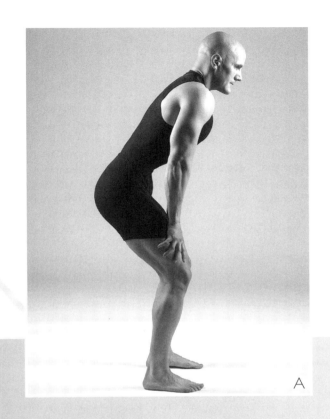

A

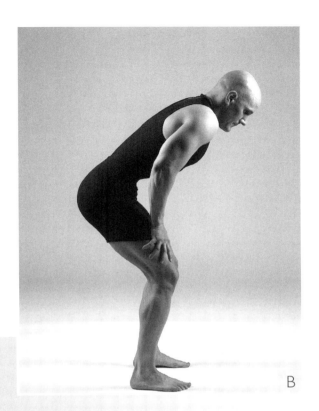

B

POSITIONS

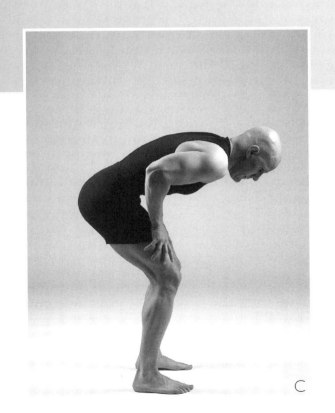

C

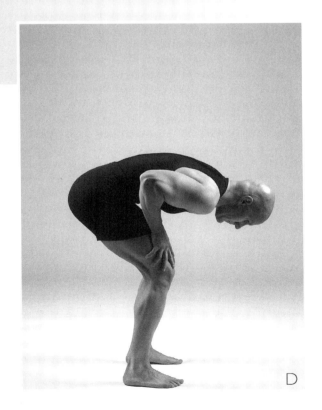

D

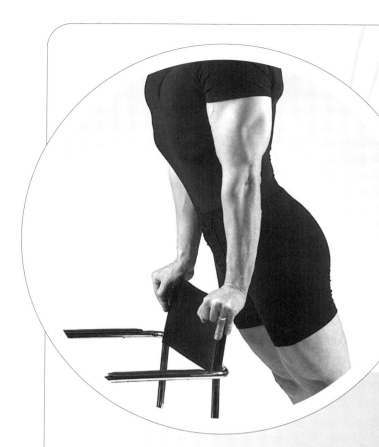

HIPS & BUTTOCKS EXERCISE #1
Hips & Buttocks Flex

Powerful hips and buttocks mean a great deal to your athletic performance, because they are used extensively in running and jumping. Whether you enjoy sprinting, long distance running, volleyball, basketball, football, martial arts, or any other sport, you need strong hips and buttocks, because this region is the source of power in the beginning of all lower body motion.

While all lower body Iso Power Flexes work this region to some extent, the following exercise focuses directly on these important muscles.

HIPS & BUTTOCKS FLEX: While holding the back of a chair for balance, stand on your toes and lean slightly forward. Begin to inhale deeply for 3 to 4 seconds as you powerfully contract the muscles of your hips and buttocks. Upon reaching peak contraction, begin a slow controlled exhalation for 7 to 12 seconds while making an *f-f-f-f* or *s-s-s-s* sound and maintaining the contraction as intensely as possible. Upon completion, relax. Power breathe for 7 to 10 breaths, and move to Iso Power Flex for the Thighs.

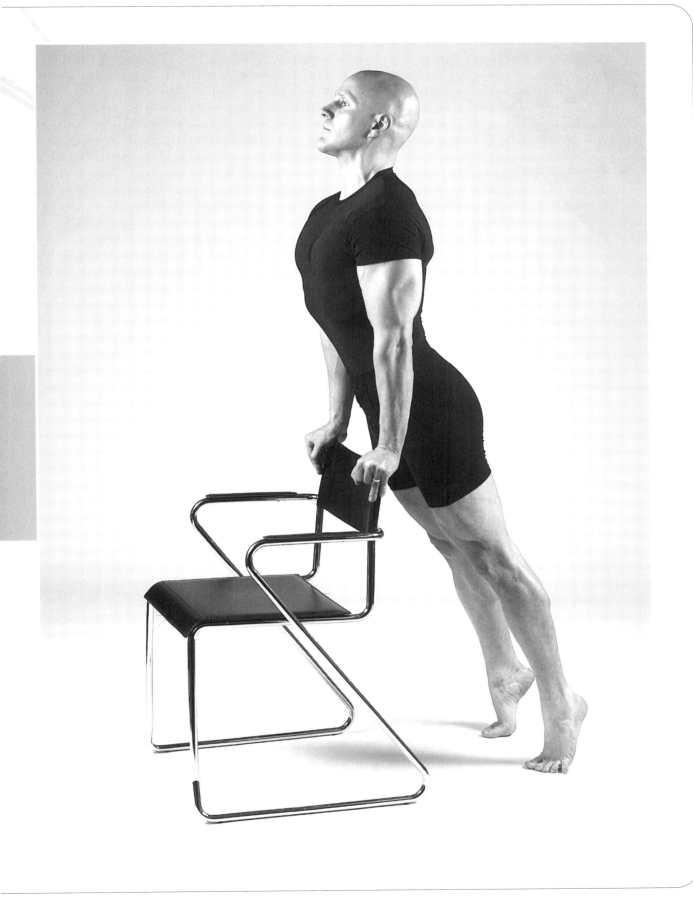

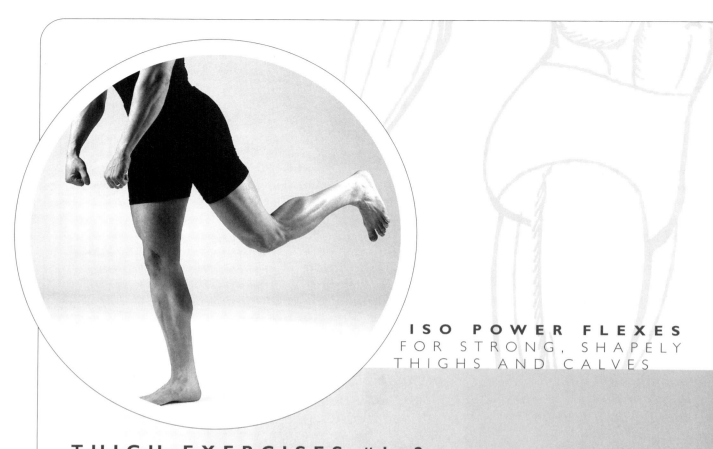

THIGH EXERCISES #1–2
Thigh Power Flexes #1–2

This section will complete your Iso Power Flex Exercises for the specific muscle groups. We have covered your entire body. This section will explain how to develop your thighs and calves.

As with the other exercises you have already learned, these exercises call upon the muscle structure of other parts of the body that come into play. For instance, you will also be working the muscles of your feet in these exercises. For anyone who wants strong, beautifully shaped thighs and calves, these exercises deliver and carry none of the risks of spinal compression or knee injury that would be caused by the use of heavy weights to accomplish the same goal. For that reason alone, Iso Power Flex is vastly superior for safe, lifelong development of the thighs and calves.

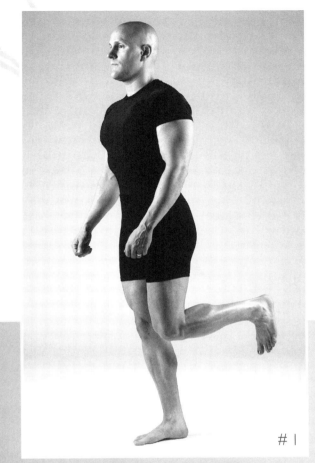

THE CRANE #1

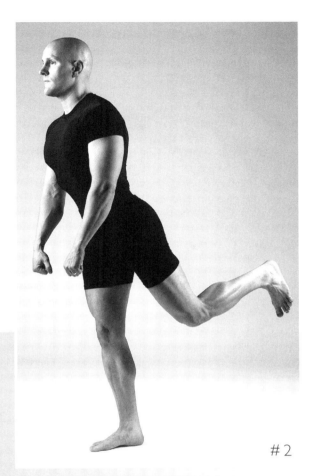

THE SWAN #2

THIGH POWER FLEX #1: Stand with your legs together. While inhaling deeply for 3 to 4 seconds, slowly lift your heel while bending the knee toward your right buttock and flex your thigh biceps as powerfully as possible. Upon reaching peak contraction, hold for 7 to 12 seconds while making an *f-f-f-f* or *s-s-s-s* sound and maintaining the contraction as intensely as possible. Upon completion, relax. Power breathe for 7 to 10 breaths, and repeat with left leg.

THIGH POWER FLEX #2: Stand with your legs together. While inhaling deeply for 3 to 4 seconds, slowly lift your right leg away from your body while slightly bending at the knee. Pull the entire leg back and up and tense as powerfully as possible (yes, you will need to lean forward). Upon reaching peak contraction, begin a slow, controlled exhalation for 7 to 12 seconds while making an *f-f-f-f* or *s-s-s-s* sound and maintaining the maximum contraction the entire time. Upon completion, relax. Power breathe for 7 to 10 breaths, and repeat with left leg.

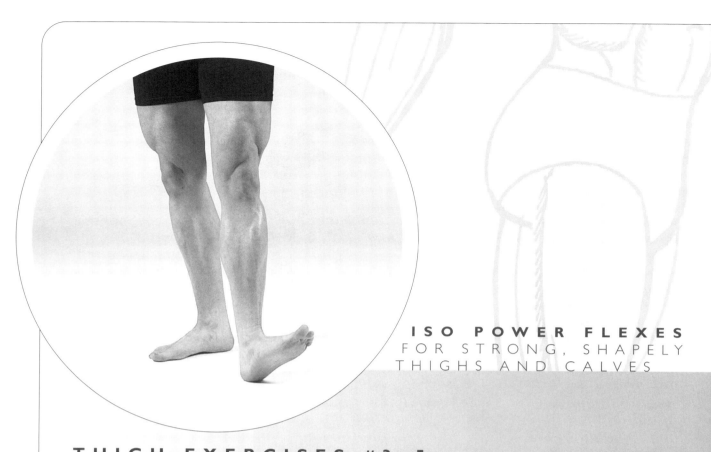

THIGH EXERCISES #3–5

Thigh Power Flexes #3–5

The next 3 Iso Power Flex Contractions are performed one leg at a time in 3 positions. The breathing, contraction, and relaxation protocols are the same for each position. Only the foot position changes.

Each exercise begins with a deep inhalation for 3 to 4 seconds while powerfully contracting the muscles. Hold at peak contraction for 7 to 12 seconds while making an *f-f-f-f* or *s-s-s-s* sound and maintaining the maximum contraction the entire time. Upon completion, relax. Power breathe for 7 to 10 breaths, and then perform the same contraction with the opposite foot.

THIGH POWER FLEX #3: Your toes are raised straight ahead; your heel is on the floor, and your knees are locked.

THIGH POWER FLEX #4: With your leg slightly in front of your body, twist your foot to the left and raise your toes as high as possible while keeping your heel down and knee locked.

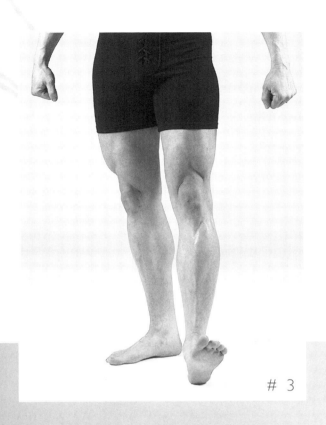

3

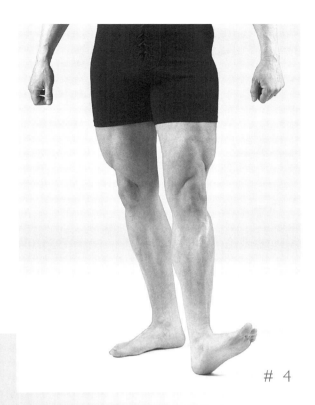

4

THIGH POWER FLEX #5: With your leg slightly in front of your body, twist your foot to the right and raise your toes as high as possible. Keep your heel on the ground, knee locked, and flex as powerfully as possible following the correct breathing and relaxation protocols.

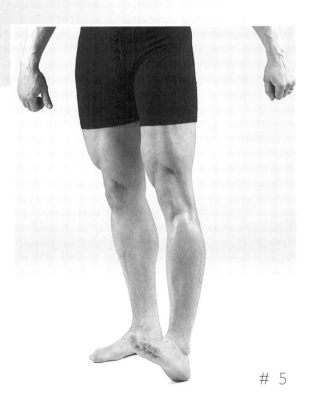

5

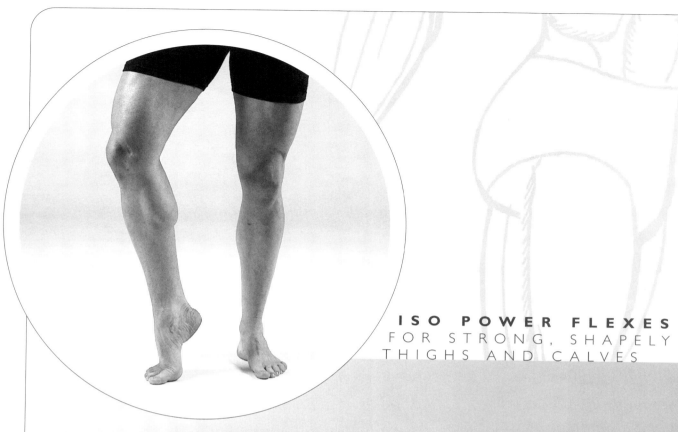

CALF EXERCISES #1–3

Calf Power Flexes #1–3

There are 5 separate contractions for the calves. Once again, only the positions change. The breathing, contraction, and relaxation protocols are identical for each.

Each exercise begins with a deep inhalation for 3 to 4 seconds while powerfully contracting the muscles. Hold at peak contraction for 7 to 12 seconds while making an *f-f-f-f* or *s-s-s-s* sound and maintaining the maximum contraction the entire time. Upon completion, relax. Power breathe for 7 to 10 breaths, and then perform the same contraction with the opposite foot.

CALF POWER FLEX #1: Stand with your right leg slightly bent at the knee, with your heel raised as high as possible. Flex your calf muscles as hard as possible. Relax. Repeat with your left leg.

CALF POWER FLEX #2: Stand with your right leg slightly bent at the knee, with your toes pointing left. Raise your heel as high as possible while tensing your calf muscles as intensely as possible. Relax. Repeat with your left leg.

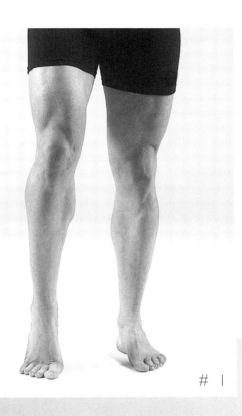

#1

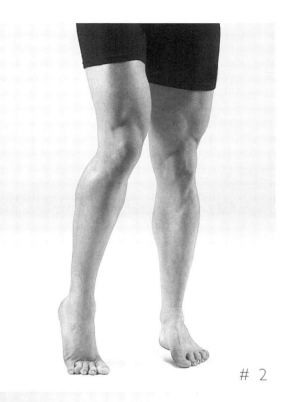

#2

CALF POWER FLEX #3: Stand with your right leg slightly bent at the knee, with your toes pointing right. Raise your heel as high as possible while tensing your calf muscles as intensely as possible. Relax. Repeat with your left leg.

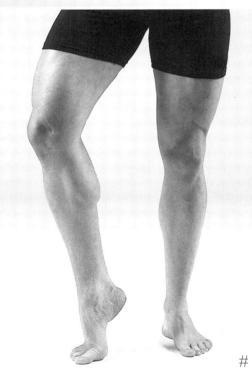

#3

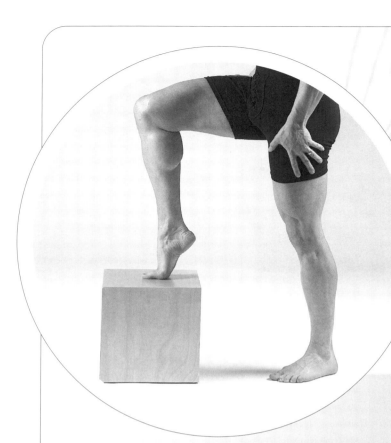

ISO POWER FLEXES
FOR STRONG, SHAPELY
THIGHS AND CALVES

CALF EXERCISES #4–5

Calf Power Flexes #4–5

CALF POWER FLEX #4: Place your right leg on a box or stool. Raise up your toes, flexing your calf muscles as intensely as possible while lifting your heel as high as possible. Relax. Repeat with your left leg.

NOTE: you may wish to change positions of your foot as previously. The choice is yours.

CALF POWER FLEX #5: Place your right leg on a box or stool and raise up your toes as high as possible while your heel remains down. Flex as powerfully as possible. Relax. Repeat with your left leg.

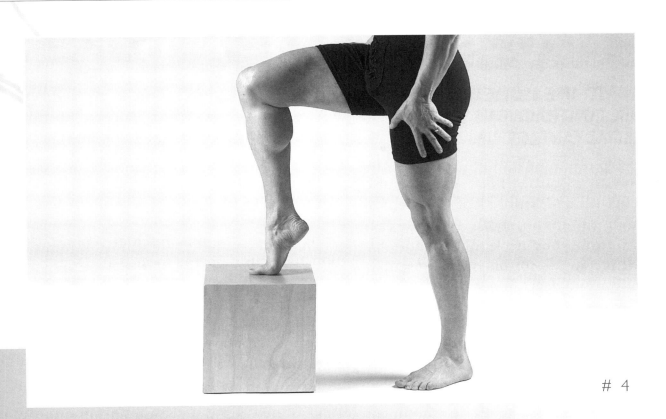

4

POSITIONS

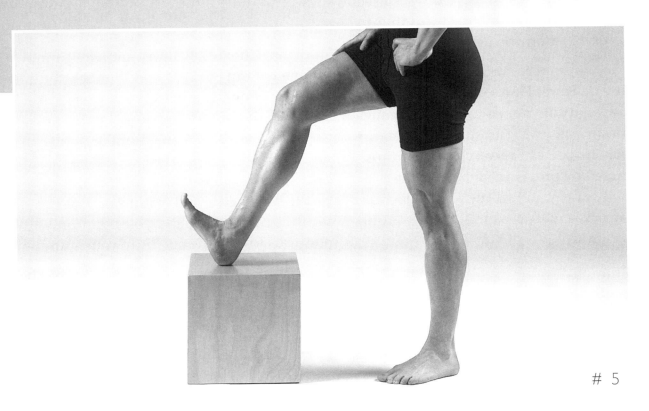

5

MUST READ!

HOW TO USE ISOMETRIC POWER FLEX CONTRACTIONS TO YOUR BEST ADVANTAGE

In Chapter 7, we featured 100 Classic Isometric Contractions that would strengthen and sculpt all of your body's muscle groups on both sides of the body from your neck to your toes at multiple angles for maximal muscular strength and development.

Having gone through Chapter 8, you have learned an additional 56 Isometric Power Flex Contractions that rely solely on contracting your muscles as powerfully as possible at their greatest angle of "pull" or contraction. Both methods yield extraordinary results and can be used either separately or blended together in any combination you desire.

If, for instance, you choose to use Isometric Power Flexes separately, you will be flexing your muscles to their maximum limit and assuming postures that are in some instances very close to those assumed by professional bodybuilders in their posing routines. The results that can be achieved with this method are nothing less than sensational.

In fact, famed bodybuilder Arnold Schwarzenegger stated in his book *The Education of a Bodybuilder* that for several weeks before a contest he didn't lift weights at all. Rather, he practiced "posing" and flexing his muscles as powerfully as possible in front of a mirror to bring out maximum muscular separation and definition and to shed all traces of body fat. That, my friend, is Isometric Power Flexing just as you have learned in this chapter, and you can accomplish the same objective by mastering these 56 featured Isometric Power Flexes.

So why is it that these Isometric Power Flexes have such a powerful effect? Because these exercises don't just stretch your muscles. They literally infuse blood into those unused fibers deep in the center of your muscles. Believe me, no gym equipment can possibly work a muscle the way your mind can. Plus, these exercises protect your joints, tendons, and ligaments and cause no spinal compression of any kind. That means they are the perfect anti-aging exercises for a lifetime of health, strength, and youthful vitality. Practice them daily, and you'll not only add years to your life but life to your years.

ACKNOWLEDGMENTS

My appreciation to my friend and director of literary development for Bronze Bow Publishing, Lance Wubbels, and my friend and chief designer, Gregory Rohm, for their consistent support, encouragement, feedback, and faith. They, along with my friends and business partners, Dave Koechel and Duff Smith, have taught me that "No one is smarter than all of us together."

SPECIAL THANKS TO:

My wife, Denise, for her love, undying support, and belief in me. For being mine and for constantly reviewing unpolished drafts of this manuscript.

My photographer, Tom Henry, for using his incredible artistic gifts on my behalf. You're incredible, Tom.

Dr. Neal Eslinger, for proving firsthand the power of the methods we teach, and for the superb job of modeling the various Isometric Power Flex Exercises. Thanks, Doc. I love you big time.

Our Bronze Bow forum members, who literally prove each day the truth of "One for All, All for One," and for being examples to the world.

To Gordan Anderson, physical culture historian, for his friendship and mentorship. I'm truly grateful.

To Roger Fillary and Gil Waldron in grateful appreciation for all their generous contributions to physical culture and especially for the website, www.sandowplus.co.uk.

To my Lord and Savior Jesus Christ, for saving me and bringing me opportunities beyond my dreams.

And, finally, my deepest thanks to all my past teachers, students, and other sources of inspiration, who are too numerous to name, but who are now a part of me.

Thanks to all of you.

John E. Peterson

From: Joris Schlötz, The Netherlands

I'm 30 years old and live in the Netherlands. I worked out with weights since I was 22, but a year ago I had to give up training because of a shoulder and back injury I sustained during training. In May 2006, I came across John Peterson's *Pushing Yourself to Power* and began practicing the Transformetrics™ techniques diligently (with some skepticism at first). To my delight, I noticed a definite increase in muscle mass after having been on the system for a mere three weeks!

However, it wasn't until a few days ago that I really became a convert. Some of my friends invited me to join them for a workout in the gym. To my absolute astonishment, I was not only able to bench press and lift the same weights I had used when I was in my weight training prime, I could even crank it up a notch and train with weights that had been beyond my limit. My friends were shocked as well. Until that moment they had never taken my "weight free" workout seriously.

I was a little worried that I had pushed it a bit too far in the gym, but I didn't experience any muscle ache or soreness. I am truly amazed by what the Transformetrics™ system has done for me. In only 4 to 5 months I reached a level of fitness that 7 years of weight training couldn't deliver. My only regret is that I didn't discover Transformetrics™ sooner.

testimonial **#2**

From: Reverend Barry Hobson, United Kingdom

I am 49 years old, and before I adopted John's training methods I lifted weights for many years. I had tried every workout system under the sun, but in reality my health and physique were in decline. I suffered from a variety of muscle/tendon problems, which were exacerbated by years of macho weight training.

Since I discovered Transformetrics™, I have been rejuvenated. I even have my old drive back to believe that I can achieve new things. For example, I now train almost every day and feel I am in control of my training and am not stuck on some preordained weight that I have to lift no matter what. The evidence for this is that since I have been practicing this protocol I have gained in both size and strength. In fact, I feel a bit silly. What is a 49-year-old man doing believing he can set new strength and health targets he failed to achieve when he was younger? Truth is, this stuff simply WORKS.

From: Edward Yah, Republic of Singapore

I started exercising about a year ago and gave up almost immediately. As a child, I was not into sports and lived a sedentary life. Whenever I started exercising, I wondered if I was doing the exercises correctly, how I should progress, and why I didn't see the results I desired. All those questions added to my frustration and despair. In high school, my physical education teacher gave up on me and said, "What good are you? You can't even carry your own body weight!"

When I discovered Bronze Bow and the Transformetrics™ training system on the Internet, the fact that I could do the exercises at home was appealing. I felt so awkward in a gym and was concerned that people would laugh at me. I discovered that the Transformetrics™ system was easy to learn and do. The books *Pushing Yourself to Power* and *The Miracle Seven* were indeed a godsend. I read the books intently and told myself the Tiger Moves were absolutely doable. For the first time I discovered the joy of working out without feeling sore all over.

And, fortunately for me, the friendship and encouragement I found on the Bronze Bow forum helped me keep going no matter how I felt. I started doing the Tiger Moves every day at slightly higher tension, and within a week I mastered the basic ability to control the muscles in my chest that I didn't even know were controllable! That gave me great encouragement, and I continued. After the second week, I began to see slight improvement in muscle definition all over my body, and my muscles felt harder and tougher. I was exhilarated, and my confidence soared.

I decided it was time to overcome a power calisthenics that had always terrified and disappointed me—the push-up! I was pleasantly surprised that after only 3 weeks of Tiger Moves, I could complete my first 6 reps of push-ups! This reinforced the endless possibilities that the Transformetrics™ training system offered, and I felt good about it in every way. To say I was highly motivated was an understatement!

Last month, doing 10 reps in a set, I continued doing sets throughout the day and accomplished 100 reps in a single day. Going from 0 to 100 push-ups per day may not be a monumental accomplishment for many people, but it is something of a miracle for me.

Since learning the Bronze Bow principle, I have never looked back...and now I'm looking forward to the day when I can accomplish what John Peterson, the most important role model in my life thus far, advocates—the ultimate *Trinity of Health and Fitness.*

I am a 40-year-old Swiss physician, who started exercising regularly 7 years ago. I used to run and cycle regularly and thought I was in good shape. Three years ago I started Krav Maga, an Israeli self-defense system, but quickly realized my body was globally out of shape. I couldn't even do a push-up, and when I tried to kick, I lost my balance and sometimes fell over. Before this, I was proud of my ability to run for 2 hours straight, even though I had an unreasonable amount of abdominal fat. One of the other practitioners used to make fun of me: "What are you doing here? Look at you. You have no chest and no arms."

With my profession and 4 children to father, I needed a system I could use at home after 10 o'clock. I surfed the Internet and ended up ordering *Pushing Yourself to Power* and began creating different routines from the exercises in that book. Then I got *The Miracle Seven* and started to do the Tiger Moves regularly. Recently, I bought the *Trinity of Health and Fitness* DVD and did the three exercises almost exclusively for 3 weeks with great results. This DVD even got my 10-year-old daughter started on doing the exercises almost every night.

For the past 3 years I have been exercising every day for at least 1 hour with the Transformetrics™ methods, changing routines frequently. Recently, my wife said I was the only man of my age without a sagging belly! I have progressed a lot in my martial art, and my teacher has asked me what I was doing to transform my physique. The other practitioner went from being critical to saying he would like to look like I do now. This summer we went camping for a few days in a tent. No problem. Every evening I did the Tiger Moves and a few other exercises outside the tent.

Your system has been a lifesaver. My energy levels are high all day. I can play with my children and carry the smaller ones for long distances without strain. I exercise at home every evening in the same room as my wife. If the children need me, I am there. Before I would be gone from the house in the evening for 2 hours at the gym. I am so pleased to have found Transformetrics™. I don't even want to imagine what my life would be like without them.

John Peterson is the KING of Isometric and body weight training. My physique has improved remarkably since I met John. Applying his vast knowledge about using your body to achieve maximum gains in muscular size, strength, and definition, I am in the best shape of my life…at 38 years old!

From: *Matt Gunther, New Jersey, USA*

I am 42 years old and have been a consistent and disciplined practitioner of Transformetrics™ for about a year now, and my transformation continues to evolve. The funny thing for me is I'm lighter now than I've ever been (about 175 pounds), but I'm much stronger and actually have better definition than when I was at 190 pounds. I can perform 10 pull-ups, which I could never do until I started using the exercises in *Pushing Yourself to Power.*

The real beauty of John's program is that you can devise your own exercise program, using it anywhere and anytime. This is great for a busy person such as me. A lot of people ask me what exercises I do, and I tell them about Transformetrics™. In my opinion, this program could put a lot of health clubs out of business.

From: *Henry Marczak, Ontario, Canada*

I first realized the benefits of calisthenics when I started Tai Chi Chuan back in 1979. I was amazed at how strong and muscular my legs got, and since then I have exercised regularly. I never got into bodybuilding, but I did start to use a home weights set in 1984. In 2000, I came down with pneumonia and had a huge cyst in my right lung, and I got so weak I could barely stand up. The doc set me up with a surgeon who was going to remove the lung, but instead I gave acupuncture a try, and it helped.

About the same time, I received the famous Charles Atlas Dynamic Tension Course. I originally had the course in 1970, but I didn't have the discipline to stick with it. This time, however, I was excited about it, and all the exercises made sense. And, yes, I fully recovered from my lung illness.

Eventually I got copies of *Pushing Yourself to Power* and *The Miracle Seven*. These books are great and have given me more scope to work with. In 2005, I took up Aikido, a modern Japanese martial art, and then got a job on a building site, where I badly strained both my arms. The only exercises I could do were the non-apparatus methods I had been learning. Pull-ups were impossible, and I still struggle with them but practice them often from wooden beams at work. Push-ups were a regular drill, and I also discovered the true power of Isometrics. Isometrics are the workingman's best friend, and doing Aikido four times a week doesn't allow for the use of weights.

Transformetrics™ is the way. Everybody's doing it.

I'm 36 years old and live in Battle Creek, Michigan. While I wasn't an elite athlete as a youth, I participated in sports and was active with my friends. But when I went to college and was working fulltime, my exercise time quickly diminished.

When I was 25, I enrolled in a martial arts school. That kept me busy, with learning and practicing the movements. Still, I wanted to increase my strength, which the martial arts alone did not help me accomplish. So, for years I played around with different routines and joined a couple local gyms. But the gym environment didn't help me get into the condition I wanted. And all those hours in the gym took away from my practice of martial arts, so I quit the gym.

I searched the Internet for "non-equipment"-based workouts and was surprised to find many sources. But there were few that actually met my criteria for no equipment. Eventually I came upon John Peterson's *Pushing Yourself to Power,* but I just couldn't grasp the concept of "Dynamic Visual Resistance" at the time. I was already experimenting with what I now refer to as "dynamic self-resistance" exercises, so I stayed with what I knew and enjoyed.

A couple years later, I found Bronze Bow Publishing and its Internet forum. I was one of the many forum members who preordered *The Miracle Seven* book. To say I was impressed with what I received is an understatement. I immediately began practicing the Tiger Moves, starting with one set of 10 reps of each move, because that amount tired me out. However, the results I achieved were amazing and fast. And, what's better is that I never experienced the typical muscle soreness I got with weights.

I soon noticed my sports jacket fit tighter, especially under the arms. And within a few months I noticed I had to tighten my belt another notch, as my waistline was decreasing. I attribute this to my performance of the "Abdominal Contraction." Recently, I traveled out of town for a conference. It's the first time I've ever been able to work out when I wasn't home.

I have a desk job, so finding a system of exercises I can do anytime, anywhere has definitely been a blessing. Whenever I hear someone talk about wanting to start working out, I mention Bronze Bow and its many publications. I don't see how a person can go wrong there. Now, the only resistance workout I do is Transformetrics™-based. I thank God and John Peterson for the development of Transformetrics™. My only regret is that I didn't find this system earlier.

From: Cliff Arceneaux, Alabama, USA

I am a 32-year-old physician assistant, who lifted weights on and off for many years. I did whatever the muscle magazines told me to do. I found some personal identity in lifting heavy amounts of iron to the awe of others. Then I herniated two lumbar discs in my back, my shoulder had its days of pain, and a torn tendon in my knee would be aggravated with squats. Then I tore a ligament in my wrist when the weight wobbled while I was benching with two 90-pound dumbbells.

During the summer 2005, budget cuts forced me to dump my cherished but only used once-a-week gym membership. So I started playing around with body weight exercises and tried some books and programs that I didn't like. I saw *Pushing Yourself to Power* on Amazon.com and read some good reviews. My wife liked the fact that the book was cheaper than a kettlebell, so with a hefty amount of skepticism and hope we bought it.

After one workout, I was sold. I was amazed that I could get a great workout at home without equipment and achieve the same "pump" I got from weights. These workouts require a new kind of strength, a tougher one than I used in lifting iron. It requires a focus and intensity I had not used in my previous training. After only 2 weeks of using the Transformetrics™ workout, my wife commented, "Your muscles look bigger."

I've been working out consistently for a year now, which is something of a personal record by itself. Usually I would have hurt myself by now and had to recover or just gotten too bored. My shoulder and wrist feel great, and the torn patellar tendon in my knee is no longer a problem. The Transformetrics™ system is built to heal and prevent injuries, promoting consistency. And consistency is the real difference between a good training system and a great one.

I look better, feel better, and am stronger than ever. I recently tested my strength at the gym and was thrilled with the results. I have increased in strength, not just maintained. For instance, having been stuck just barely benching my body weight, I can now bench well over that for solid reps with no problems. Whoo-hoo!

I am thankful to John Peterson and the Bronze Bow forum members for continuing to teach me that "You Are Your Own Gym."

I am 58 years old and fortunate to be alive. I have degenerative joint disease from head to toe, which probably started years ago when I was almost killed by a drunk driver who hit my car head-on. My family doctor worked on me in the emergency room that night and couldn't recognize me because my face was so messed up. Besides numerous other injuries, I lost the sight in my left eye due to the accident. A later car accident, where I was hit by a car going 100 miles an hour, gave me a fractured sternum and dislocated thumbs. In all, I've had 52 surgeries, including 2 cervical fusions, tendons and ligaments stapled to my shoulder to prevent dislocation, a collarbone cut out due to injury, surgery on my lower back for a herniated L-4 disc, and numerous other fusions.

Last year my daughter had to rush me to the emergency room because I had an abscess on my intestines that burst, and I had to have a foot of my intestine removed. I had complications from that surgery and couldn't work for 7 months. My weight shot up to 188 pounds, and I'm only 5'1". That extra weight made my joint pain worse. I couldn't walk across the room without having chest pain, and my pulse would shoot up to 132 or higher. I felt as though I was going to pass out. My doctor wanted me in the hospital for fear of a possible heart attack or stroke, but I couldn't afford it. I'm on disability income and work 15 hours a week at a video store for minimum wage.

I was desperate and scared. I decided one day to try to speak with John Peterson. I told him what was going on, and he listened patiently and then told me something that changed my life. He said that despite my joint pain, I could still do Isometrics. After I hung up, I had a choice to make—either continue on as I was or I could try to do something about it. I decided to take John's advice and set out to get better. I found a way to modify my body weight exercises to lessen the pain, did *The Miracle Seven* exercises, and focused on Isometrics. After 3 months I had lost 32 pounds and looked as good as I did when I was in my twenties! My customers at the video store all ask me what in the world I did to change. I tell them about *Pushing Yourself to Power* and *The Miracle Seven* plus Isometrics!

The point is that if these methods can produce results in a busted up 57-year-old man like me, just think of the results it can have if you're healthy. One phone call changed my life, and I am living proof that John Peterson's methods can change your life as well.

ANYTIME. ANYWHERE. TOTAL STRENGTH & FITNESS FOR MEN & WOMEN.

Imagine a complete strength and fitness program that slims, shapes, and sculpts your entire body in just 20 minutes a day. A program you can do anytime and virtually anywhere. A program so complete it requires no gym and no exercise equipment. Best of all, a program that covers every muscle group from your neck to your toes and delivers visible results in as little as 3 weeks.

Using the revolutionary Transformetrics™ Training System that utilizes time-tested body sculpting techniques along with high-tension Isometrics that literally allow you to become your own gym, *The Miracle Seven* offers:

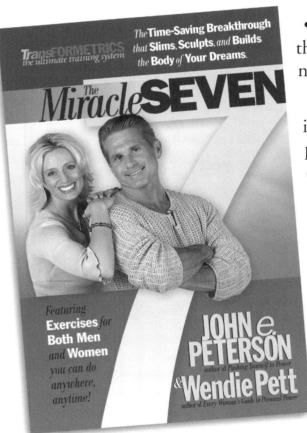

• A 20-minute per day weekly plan that sculpts the entire body to its own natural perfection.

• Detailed day-by-day exercise instruction, fully illustrated with photos that show each and every exercise.

• A special "speed it up" program that accelerates fat-burning results for those who want to see their results yesterday.

• A comprehensive nutrition plan that allows you to lose body fat faster than you gained it while providing easy to follow guidelines for eating healthy.

• The exhilaration that comes from knowing that you have complete control over your body, your life, and your destiny!

 Available at **www.bronzebowpublishing.com**

IF YOU'VE BEEN LOOKING FOR AN EXERCISE SYSTEM that will give you the results you've always dreamed of having, does not require either a gym or expensive exercise equipment, can be done anytime and anyplace without requiring an outrageous commitment of time, you're holding it in your hands.

Based solidly upon the most effective exercise systems as taught by Earle E. Liederman and Charles Atlas during the 1920s, *Pushing Yourself to Power* provides you with everything you need to know to help your body achieve its natural, God-given strength and fitness potential. Whether your desire is simply to slim down and shape up, or to build your maximum all-around functional strength, athletic fitness, and *natural* muscularity, you will find complete training strategies specifically tailored to the achievement of your personal goals.

Precisely illustrated with 100s of clear, detailed photos showing every facet of every exercise, you'll never have to guess if you're doing it right again. You'll achieve the stamina you've always wanted in less time than it requires to drive to a gym and change into exercise clothes. Feel what it's like to have twice as much energy as you ever thought you'd have!

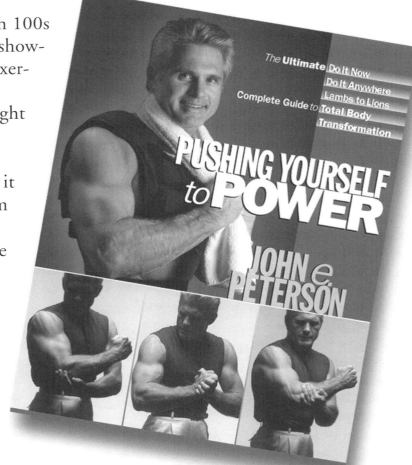

THE TRANSFORMETRICS™ TRAINING SYSTEM offers the most honest, straightforward approach to safe, lifelong strength, youthfulness, and long-term fat loss ever created. It is founded on the premise that there are no quick fixes, no magic diets, and nobody has a magic wand to give people the lithe, athletic, sculpted physique they've always dreamed of having. Three things are required: the right balance of nutritious foods, the right strength-building, body-sculpting exercise system, and the knowledge and commitment to put them together.

In the *60 Day Personal Power Health & Fitness Journal*, John and Wendie offer:

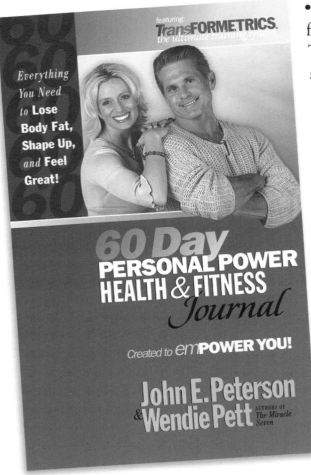

• A complete exercise program featuring the Transformetrics™ Training System to help people slim, strengthen, and help their body achieve its natural, God-given strength and fitness potential…without the requirement of a gym or expensive exercise equipment.

• Complete food charts that feature protein, fat, and carbohydrate grams as well as calories.

• User-friendly exercise charts to help people keep track of their daily progress.

• And inspiring quotes, scriptures, and more to help them stay motivated.

 Available at **www.bronzebowpublishing.com**